THE DREAM . . .
THE JOURNEY

LORAIN
COMMUNITY
HOSPITAL

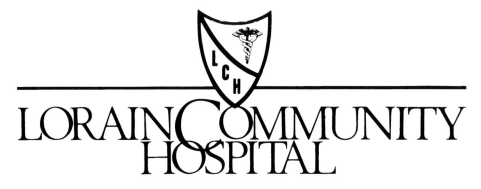

LORAIN COMMUNITY HOSPITAL

member **University Hospitals** Network

THE DREAM . . .

THE JOURNEY

LORAIN

COMMUNITY

HOSPITAL

Heritage Publishers, Inc.
Flagstaff, Arizona

THE DREAM . . .
THE JOURNEY

LORAIN
COMMUNITY
HOSPITAL

by Paul C. Balcom
as told to Margaret Finnerty

Edited by Amy Phillips
Book design by Vanessa Davisson

Heritage Publishers, Inc.
2700 Woodlands Boulevard, Suite 300
Flagstaff, Arizona 86001-7124
(602) 526-1129   (800) 972-8507

ISBN 929690-20-6
Library of Congress Cataloging Number 93-79462

Printed and bound in the United States of America

DEDICATION

This book is dedicated to the individuals who dreamed the dream and journeyed the journey and who today continue to plan for the future.

Treating each patient with individualized care, Judy Zakutny, specialized procedures technician of radiology, assists patient Diane Deedrick.

The main visitors' entrance, 1993

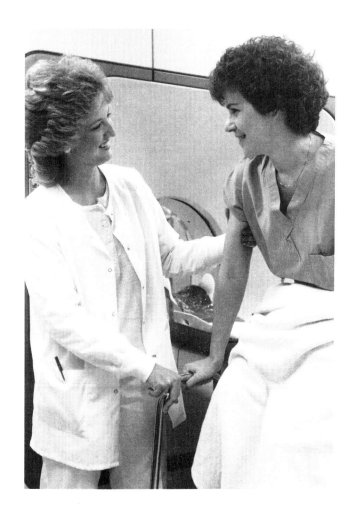

TABLE OF CONTENTS

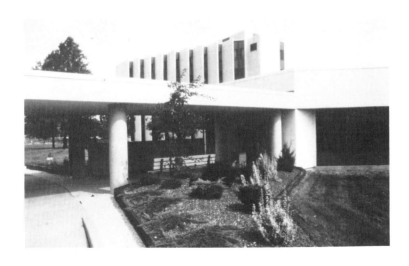

ACKNOWLEDGEMENTS

We would like to thank those whose gracious cooperation made this book possible:

The advisory committee, whose direction simplified research and speeded production of the manuscript: Paul Balcom, Stanley Pijor, Laurie Hoke, Alice Weston, and Robert Capretto

Individuals who were interviewed: Paul Balcom, Donald Blanford, M. D., Ruth Calta, Laurie Hoke, Michael Kolczun II, M. D., Denis Radefeld, M. D., Stanley Pijor, Gerald Prucha, David Ross, John Schaeffer, M. D., Vincent Traina, William Wickens, Alice Weston, and Florencio Yuzon, M. D.

Those who assisted in photo location and identification and with the inevitable "last bit of information": Becky Williams, Joan Shoop, and Mike Stoltz

The roots of this publication lie in the painstaking research and lively descriptions found in Alice Weston's early history of Lorain Community Hospital. Her initial efforts and continuing support gave color and character to this story.

Finally, we would like to extend our sincere appreciation to Paul C. Balcom, President and Chief Executive Officer of Lorain Community Hospital. Under his leadership, project meetings were short but effective, decisions were made in a timely manner, and positive guidance was always available. Mr. Balcom, thank you for making this book a reality.

The Publisher

The Dream...The Journey
Lorain Community Hospital

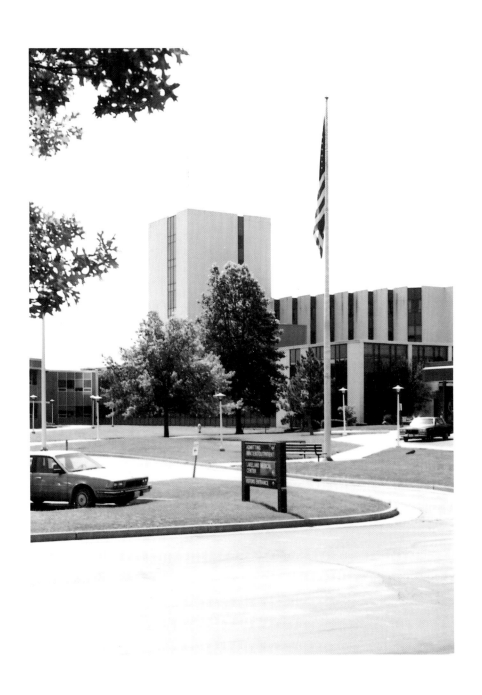

Lorain Community
Hospital, 1993

*"Inside Tree of Life,"
decorated on January 18,
1991, in honor of our men
and women called to serve
during the Persian Gulf
crisis. "Keeping Friends
and Loved Ones Close—
Though Worlds Apart."*

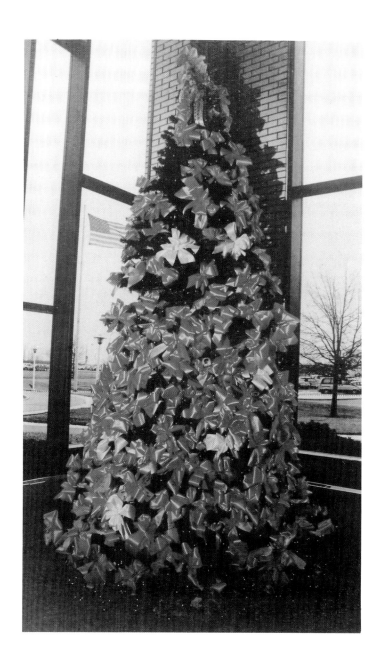

The Dream...The Journey
Lorain Community Hospital

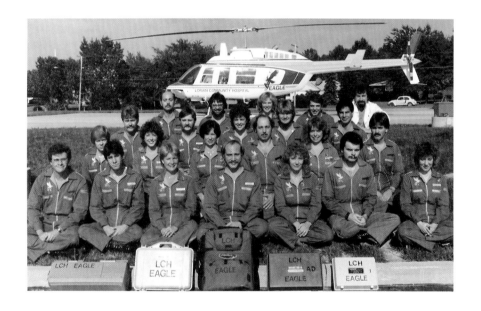

Lorain Community Hospital's EAGLE (Emergency Assistance to Ground and Lake Environments) served the community for nearly two years staffed by this team of paramedics, trauma nurses and pilots.

Preserving the precious gift of sight is the Regional Eye program at Lorain Community Hospital. Using the latest in sophisticated diagnostic services and state-of-the-art surgical techniques, the program has become a major eye service center in the region.

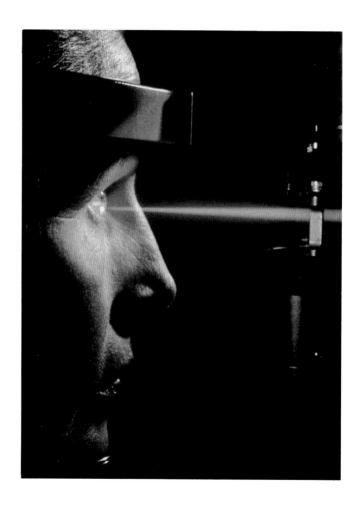

PREFACE

When we look at the spectacular health care campus that we call Lorain Community Hospital, it presents something of a puzzle. The buildings are bright and modern, yet it seems to many people as if the hospital has been here forever.

How many of us have spent time with loved ones there? How many remember tonsillectomies, or broken bones set, or perhaps coming home from the hospital following a major or minor emergency? Who hasn't spent anxious hours in one of the waiting rooms, unconsciously aware of the caring and competent people moving quietly by, intent on their healing tasks? And who has not responded to the numerous appeals to the community to help "our" hospital when a new piece of equipment or an addition to the building was needed to improve the quality of Lorain Community Hospital?

Undoubtedly, the hospital is part of our lives, part of our city. But to know the whole story, we must go back to the Eisenhower era and meet some Lorain citizens with an audacious idea.

The narrative encompasses three decades, but the real story is the one that continues today: state-of-the-art technology combined with ageless compassion to face the challenges of tomorrow.

*Angie Knittle comforts a
patient in the cardiac
catheterization
laboratory.*

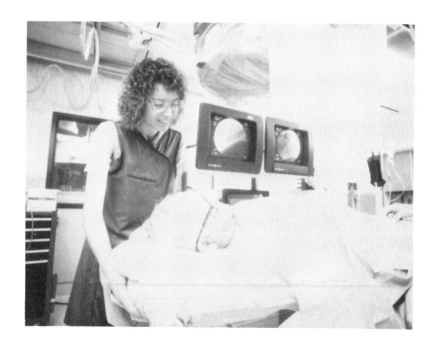

LORAIN COMMUNITY HOSPITAL
MISSION STATEMENT

Lorain Community Hospital will be recognized as a leader in identifying and evaluating health care needs of the local and regional community, and in providing a broad spectrum of selected health care services, programs, and activities in response to the needs of patients, families, institutions, payors, and health care professionals.

Our patients will receive quality health care delivered in a safe and supportive environment by skilled and caring professionals. Quality health care means understanding and meeting the requirements of those we serve, both internally and externally.

Lorain Community Hospital will be contemporary, progressive, and innovative in structuring services and in establishing relationships with other providers and consumers of health care.

Patients will be received and needed care given without regard to the patient's economic status or ability to pay, consistent with available hospital resources.

This will be accomplished within an economically viable environment while meeting our community obligations.

Approved by the
Lorain Community Hospital Board of Trustees
January 1, 1988

INTRODUCTION

The dream that made Lorain Community Hospital was only one of many dreams that became reality in the history-rich north coast of Ohio. The journey that took the hospital from conception to maturity was just one of many journeys in an area especially blessed with paths for travelers.

With its imposing physical plant, Lorain Community Hospital is an institution any city would be proud to possess. It is not only an impressive health care facility but also a major area employer and worthy corporate citizen. The community can truly share the story of how the hospital came to be.

Some would argue that the story of a town's medical care is just a footnote in a chronicle that parallels the nation's own history. But to ignore this story is to belittle the most important element in any history: the people who made things happen. These are the pioneers who create homes in the wilderness, endure natural disasters, survive economic and technological changes, and still maintain a generous human response: to make the community better.

Those who first dreamed of a fine new hospital for a growing community were the descendants—real or spiritual—of generations who lived by the lake and built their lives around it and the land it bordered. The earliest inhabitants not only fished the waters of Lake Erie and the

Black River but used them as a means of transportation. The scenic beauty and economic potential of the area must have impressed early European visitors, who passed through in the seventeenth century. Valuable for hunting and fishing, the area was the site of many battles among the native tribes, including Ottawas, Eries, Hurons, Delawares, and Chippewas. By 1745, the strategic value of the location caused the British to build a fort near Sandusky. For two decades, off and on, they clashed with French forces as well as some of the native tribes. In 1763, the Treaty of Paris ceded the disputed land to Great Britain.

The Revolution freed the American colonies, now states, from restrictions on western expansion, and in 1787, the Northwest Territory was established. Newly independent Americans were soon drawn to the mouth of the Black River. When they arrived in 1810, John S. Reid and other early settlers were attracted by the rich farmland, but they soon capitalized on the river site to build ships as well. The skills of Connecticut shipwrights Augustus Johns and William Murdock were the foundation of an industry that would continue in the area into the late twentieth century.

Lorain County was organized in 1824. Ten years later, the little settlement on the Black River declared itself the town of Charlestown.

Neighboring Cleveland was the terminus of the Ohio Canal, completed in 1832; that town's inevitable growth also attracted railroads and ore shipments in the 1850s. While this activity seemed to leave its neighbors behind, the substantial industrial boom begun during the Civil

War reached Lorain County twenty years later. The arrival of its own railroad, the Cleveland, Lorain and Wheeling, connected the area with the coal fields to the south. Charleston's substantial fishing industry would be overshadowed by heavy industry.

In 1874, an attempt to incorporate Charlestown met a snag; there was already a town with that name on the books. The town council agreed to adopt the name of their county, which had been chosen by an early pioneer who had a fondness for the French province of Lorraine.

The end of the century found Lorain a prosperous town; dredging and widening the river had attracted more industry. Steel and ships and heavy equipment provided jobs for over 5,000 residents. In 1892, St. Joseph Hospital was established to serve the town's health needs.

Town became city, as floods of immigrants sought the American dream in Lorain's factories. Hundreds of houses were built to shelter them,

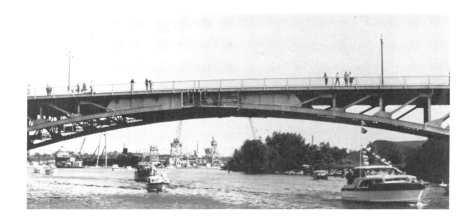

Where the Black River meets Lake Erie, Lorain Harbor. A landmark of the harbor is the bascule bridge, dedicated in 1940. Photograph courtesy of the Black River Historical Society of Lorain

as well as schools, churches, theaters, and a library. By 1902 the population
had passed 27,000.

During World War I, Lorain provided both armaments and
servicemen. The industrial expansion continued, and the population
increased, but Lorain's history was fated to take a somber turn.

For five heart-stopping minutes in the summer of 1924, a tornado
ripped through downtown Lorain, killing seventy-eight and virtually
destroying the business district. With its usual determination, the city
began to rebuild immediately, but another powerful force would cause
even more damage. The Great Depression checked economic growth
nationwide and stilled Lorain's factories.

New Deal work projects provided the few bright notes in a glum
decade. Schools and public buildings received needed repair. Lorain
achieved a degree of fame in engineering circles when the counter-
balanced bridge on Erie Avenue was completed; it was proclaimed the
second-largest bascule bridge in the world.

World War II brought forth more heroism from Lorain residents on
both home front and battle line. And victory again brought prosperity. The
1950 census revealed a population of 51,202. The city and its surrounding
areas were straining an infrastructure designed for a minor factory town.
Civic leaders were working with industrial executives to serve the needs of
an ambitious, multicultural urban population. And Lorain's women were
among those who dreamed of an even better community.

CHAPTER ONE

The Dream:
From Conception to
Ground-breaking

The Lakeland Woman's Club had reason to boast. It was a large and busy organization, with activities and committees to occupy the free hours of Lorain's women. There were committees devoted to diversions like bridge and antique-collecting, but the club's real pride came from the creation and development of long-term social programs. Following the example of active women's groups throughout American history, they addressed community problems and set their considerable energies to solving those problems. One noteworthy accomplishment of their powerful Civic and Community Affairs Department was the establishment of a local YWCA. The Young Women's Christian Association was approaching the centennial of its founding in the United States, and its programs would serve Lorain well, but this group was not the sort to rest on its laurels. What would be next?

Ruth Calta, one of the "founding mothers" and current member of the Hospital Board of Trustees, recalled that the chair of the Civic and Community Affairs Department, June Steen, suggested that the city could use another hospital. The new Ford Motor Company plant had brought many additional people to the area; U.S. Steel had employee rolls twice the total population of Lorain in 1892, when the community's first hospital was established. Over the years St. Joseph Hospital had grown, of course, but it was limited physically by its downtown location.

"Lorain was the fastest-growing community between New York and Chicago at that time," Mrs. Calta recalled. "All those people were going to need hospital care. So that was our project!"

Laurie Hoke, another "founding mother" and current member of the Hospital Board of Trustees, could also see considerable need for a second hospital. It was important, however, to back personal observation with documented public opinion. Also, community support was vital to such an undertaking.

"The way we went about it was interesting," Mrs. Hoke remembered. "Phone books were torn apart and each committee member was given a section and instructed to call every name on her pages. The city directory contained 25,068 phone numbers!

"The overwhelming response was incredible. There was a very strong feeling that we needed another hospital."

The Civic and Community Affairs Department had its new mission and a sense of the community. Its members knew the importance of enlisting powerful civic leaders to their cause.

"Up to that point it was only women," Mrs. Hoke pointed out. "The next thing to do was get greater representation of the community, specifically men. So they called a meeting at the American Legion on

The Dream: From Conception
to Groundbreaking

Westbury Avenue. Lawyers, businessmen, and all kinds of prominent people were called together." Over 200 people attended the meeting on February 25, 1957, and heard a litany of reasons why their community needed a second hospital: long waiting lists for elective surgery, dangerous waiting periods, the lack of facilities for heart-attack victims and those needing critical care. Many patients, it was pointed out, felt obliged to go as far as Cleveland for hospitalization.

A Hospital Facilities Committee was formed; prominent and willing citizens who volunteered included attorney William Wickens and businessman David Ross. Grace Standen, a trust officer at the Lorain National Bank, was elected temporary chair and secretary. A special guest at the meeting was Vernon Siefer, Executive Director of Cleveland's Fairview Hospital. He was asked to explain the steps in creating a new hospital. He told his attentive listeners that from start to finish it would take seven years before the hospital could open its doors.

Such a daunting announcement might have stunned a lesser group. Both Ruth Calta and Laurie Hoke agreed that their earlier naiveté carried them through situations wiser souls would have abandoned.

"We didn't know any differently," Mrs. Calta admitted. "We just felt the need and went out and encouraged people."

Mrs. Hoke was new to the community, and she believed that was probably one of her strong points.

"I would go where nobody else would dare to go, because I didn't know any better."

Where the women lacked personal knowledge about founding a hospital, they were quick to locate experts. For legal advice they retained a local attorney, Andrew Warhola.

Through him they hired Chicago hospital consultant Ross Garrett. His prominent firm's planning fee was $5,000. Implementing this advice would take both time and money. It would be almost three years before a suggested bond issue became a reality.

At a meeting in attorney Ray Miraldi's office, a concerned group assessed the situation. Charles Herzer, David Ross, and Andy Warhola listened as Laurie Hoke, Ruth Calta, and June Steen admitted that they didn't have that kind of money.

Mrs. Calta remembered Warhola's confidence in her group.

"He said that never before in his life had he signed a sort of blank check to a group of women who were willing to go out and get a hospital. 'I knew you could do it because of what you had done in the past; I knew the quality of women in the group.'"

Ross Garrett was no stranger to Lorain; he had recently conducted a successful improvement program for St. Joseph Hospital. His knowledge of the city's resources and potential was invaluable. According to Alice Weston, a television executive who later chronicled the history of the hospital, Garrett's advice was "to start with the city fathers and have them approve a bond issue and have it put on the ballot."

The group had already accepted responsibility for the expense of two experts. Promotion of the bond issue presented a need for additional funds. Professional fund-raising was not the well-known business it later became; besides, women's clubs through the ages have had their traditional methods. They moved into high gear with card parties, rummage sales, raffles, and candy sales. They held fashion shows, using their own members to model clothing supplied by downtown merchants. They took advantage of Lorain's "pennant fever" and invited wives of the Cleveland Indians baseball team members to lend luster to their fund-raisers.

The efforts were sincere, and the work was hard, yet over two years the committee had raised a painfully small war chest.

If the history of Lorain Community Hospital is ever translated to the silver screen, at this point Judy Garland would tell Micky Rooney, "I know how we can raise the money! We'll have a show! We can use Grandpa's barn!"

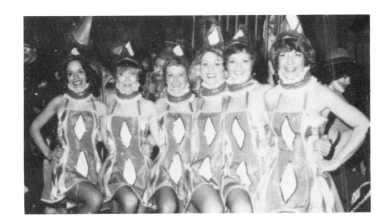

The LCH Follies is a bi-annual fund-raiser that means fun for the entire community. Year after year, residents of Lorain turn out to see friends and family flaunt their talents.

When Laurie Hoke heard about a new kind of money-making idea, she knew just the group that could and would do it. "That's how the Follies started. Of course, that's where we made our big money." The idea of a benefit performance was an attractive one, especially when, as Alice Weston recalled, "Jerome Cargill came to Lorain from New York and told the women they could put on a follies with local people, and he could guarantee they would make $10,000." His enthusiasm won over the committee, and soon one hundred local "stars" and fifty temporary "stagehands" were performing under the direction of the professionals provided by Jerome H. Cargill Productions. Everyone else in town was queuing for the five-dollar tickets, which allowed them into the Lorain High School auditorium to enjoy their neighbors' previously undiscovered talents.

True to the prophecy, in three evenings in October 1960, the show raised $10,000, far outstripping every other project's returns.

At the same time the Follies were in rehearsal, the Hospital Bond Issue Campaign Committee was planning strategies to guarantee victory at the polls. This task was not as easy as the popular sentiment for the hospital suggested.

"Everything we did at that time became controversial—absolutely everything!" Laurie Hoke recalled.

Traditional loyalty to the existing hospital caused some to view building a new hospital in religious terms. Though emotions were heated, in reality there were supporters of every religion on both sides.

The Dream: From Conception
to Groundbreaking

A second issue that caused friction was the matter of osteopathic physicians. Though their training was different from that of mainstream physicians and surgeons, a large number of D. O.s (doctors of osteopathy) practiced in the Lorain area. Many labor unions sided with the osteopathic physicians.

The hospital matter had become truly political by the introduction of Proposition 12, the bond issue, into the 1960 ballot. And in Lorain, as in many American cities, local politics not only pitted Democrats against Republicans but also divided the city into camps along lines of ethnic, economic, religious, and labor-management loyalties. In addition to local issues, voter interest was high that year because of the exciting presidential race between Richard Nixon and John Kennedy.

On election day, when the smoke cleared, the hospital bond issue had passed by a formidable 70.3 percent—the highest percentage of any

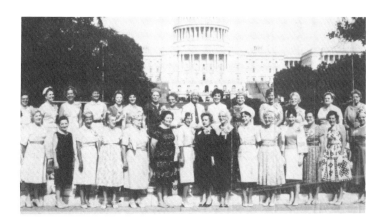

In 1963, women of the Civic and Community Affairs Department of the Lakeland Woman's Club traveled to Washington, D. C., to compete in the Sears, Roebuck scrapbook contest. Top row (left to right): Charlotte Clarke, Ruth Calta, Jean Cox, Jean Fenton, Rose Grego, Carol Dickason, Agnes Pratsch, Lucy Shreffler, Bud Lockhart (bus driver), Rita Hawley, Vi Henry, Lois Schulz, Nell Deidrick, Vera Goodell, Emma Pratsch Bottom row: Sally Bobel, Lou Kepler, Mary Newman, Grace Bumbaugh, Nellie Love, Clara Clark, Hazel Torbert, Maxine Hoak, Dorothy Schmidt, Jo Smith, Laurie Hoke, Ida Kress, Eleanor Novello, Grace Reynolds, Elva Young, June Steen.

11

---

issue in the history of Lorain elections.

The next step, according to state law, required the mayor to appoint a five-member Hospital Commission. Mayor John Jaworski named Ruth Calta, Steve Szuhy, Leo Svete, and Lewis Goodell, and took an ex officio seat himself. They promptly engaged Ross Garrett to continue in his role as consultant, and Warren and Jean Finkel as architects.

The selection of a site was an important one. The new facility had to be convenient to its patients, but in no way should it crowd the existing hospital. It should have plenty of room for expansion—but could property outside the city limits be considered? Cost could not be ignored; in addition to over a dozen properties offered for sale, the M. O'Neill Company offered a free site near its shopping center. There was some

Mayor John Jaworski and Ruth Calta at the ground-breaking, May 9, 1962. Mrs. Calta's shovel in one hand and a clipboard in the other symbolized the hard work and organization of the Civic and Community Affairs Department of the Lakeland Woman's Club.

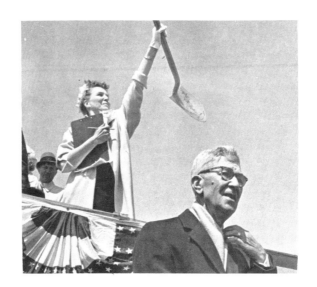

12

The Dream: From Conception
to Groundbreaking

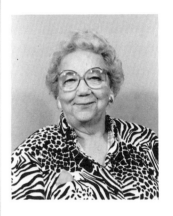

Chairman of the Community and Civic Affairs Department of the Lakeland Woman's Club, June Steen, was instrumental in seeing Lorain Community Hospital to reality.

feeling that the location near the commercial area was not ideal.

The decision was the responsibility of the Lorain City Council. On an April evening in 1961, the council voted approval of a parcel called the Kolbe Trust Property as the hospital site; it was their first formal action toward building the hospital after passage of the bond issue. The property, bounded by Kolbe Road and West Erie Avenue, had been recommended by Ross Garrett.

Fund-raising efforts continued; more money would be needed than the income raised by the bond issue. Besides a second Follies held in October, 1961, other efforts included a local ballet school's performance of Swan Lake. An unusual fund-raising effort was entering a competition sponsored by the Sears, Roebuck Company. More than 10,000 applicants nationwide submitted scrapbooks illustrating projects benefiting their communities. The Lorain Community Hospital Scrapbook was a labor of love that involved hours of research and compilation. In February, 1962, a busload of enthusiasts rode to Washington, D. C., for the awards presentation. The Lorain entry carried off third prize and a $3,000 donation for their cause.

There were a few tears of joy shed on May 9, 1962, among the forty women who had cherished a dream for five long years. They watched newly elected mayor Woodrow W. Mathna and his predecessor and political rival, former mayor John C. Jaworski, break ground at the site of the new Lorain Community Hospital. But the surreptitious tears changed to delighted laughter when they saw June Steen clamber onto a bulldozer. It seemed somehow fitting: two men ceremoniously wielding shovels (which would be duly preserved in a place of honor in the hospital's lobby) while their own representative attacked the task with heavy equipment.

THE PLAIN DEALER, TUESDAY, SEPTEMBER 15, 1964

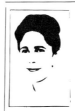

Lakeland Women Got Idea, Money for New Hospital

By DAVID KENT
Plain Dealer Bureau

LORAIN—The new Lorain Community Hospital is largely the product of 40 energetic women — members of the community and civic affairs department of Lakeland Woman's Club.

The department started intensive work in 1957 to promote a second hospital for Lorain and raised between $35,000 and $40,000 over the five years of the campaign.

BY 1962, the women had shown enough progress to be selected as third winners of an award on community achievement in a national contest with 5,000 entries.

The award by the General Federation of Women's Clubs included a $3,000 cash prize. That money also went into the hospital fund.

The intensive campaign started after a 1956 poll of all persons listed in the Lorain telephone book that showed 98% felt Lorain needed a second hospital.

YET TWO EARLIER attempts to construct a hospital—in about 1941 and 1951—had failed.

"That was probably because they didn't have enough money. Our biggest asset was that we could raise money," said Mrs. George Hoke, who was active in developing plans for the hospital as a member of the department.

Mrs. Hoke is still a member of the department and is also a member of the hospital board of trustees.

U.S. Rep. Charles A. Mosher of Ohio's 13th District thought the department's achievements so noteworthy he had a history of the battle for the hospital entered into the Congressional record.

MRS. HOKE, in an interview, stressed that apathy was the greatest initial problem the women encountered.

"But we worked on the philosophy that lots of little people can band together to move mountains to dispel the attitude of, 'Oh, I only have one little vote,'" Mrs. Hoke said.

She also said part of the success was due to the attitude of the women when they met a problem. "We didn't start throwing stones, but instead we asked these people to continue meeting with us and thereby keep the lines of communications open."

Fund-raising projects included the two largest card parties ever held in the city, rummage sales, a charity ball, a country store in downtown Lorain, a luncheon and fashion show and several stage shows.

THESE FUNDS went for initial payments for a site consultant and architect and paid all the promotion expenses of a $3.5-million bond issue that appeared on the general election ballot in 1960.

During the bond issue campaign, the women again reverted to a telephone campaign and called each of the 30,458 registered voters urging their support of the bond issue.

Apparently the voters listened because the bond issue got a whopping 70.1% favorable vote—the largest majority vote ever recorded in Lorain history.

"IT WAS TRULY miraculous that the community had supported the new hospital so overwhelmingly when it would mean taxation at a time when Lorain had made national headlines, because it was considered a depressed area due to the high percentage of unemployment," the Congressional Record reprint said.

Mrs. Hoke did not seem to be overwhelmed by the feat of the women. She explained that women's groups can do things if they want to do them badly enough—"If they have a burning desire and feel a close identification with the project."

CHAPTER TWO

Making It Happen:
A Hospital is Born

Though the hospital was seven years from idea to opening, Ruth
Calta insists that the group never gave in to discouragement. "Not once.
We even added more women to the group."

The joyous ground-breaking in May of 1962 was an inevitable, if
not immediate, result of the earlier triumph of the 1960 bond issue. The
challenges that created the lag between the original idea of a second
hospital and the passage of the bond issue that would finance it did not
disappear after election day.

One major obstacle had been the question of osteopaths. When the
science of osteopathy was founded by Dr. Andrew Tayor Still in 1874, it
was based on the manipulation of parts of the body for the prevention and
treatment of disease. For several years, area practitioners had considered
building an osteopathic hospital, since they were not allowed to treat their
patients in most local hospitals. More than a decade before the women's
group started their quest, a hard-working group had formed the Lorain
General Hospital Association. Attorney William Wickens drew up articles
of incorporation for them.

"It was a paper corporation, and it was chartered by the state," he recalled. With door-to-door solicitations, they had raised some money to help make the osteopathic facility a reality, but the plan was eventually derailed due to lack of sufficient funds. The contributions were prudently invested in hopes of some future opportunity. In the meantime, Lorain Community Hospital had become a possibility, and the osteopathic physicians were understandably bitter about yet another hospital being planned without their input. They felt sure they would not be allowed to practice in such a hospital.

The American Medical Association had opposed hospitals with "open staff," citing the differences in training and standards. They usually refused accreditation to such hospitals, which eliminated teaching courses and AMA recognition of internships and residencies. The AMA did concede that, in rare cases where local law required open staffing, dual practice was possible.

Weeks of serious negotiations between the two medical groups, M. D.s and D. O.s, seemed to be fruitless. Ross Garrett, at one point, described a hospital in California that was served by both kinds of doctors; they worked on opposite sides of a brick wall. Perhaps the absurdity of this example helped bring about compromise. All area D. O.s were invited to join the as-yet-nonexistent staff of Lorain Community Hospital. In exchange, they and their supporters would back the $3.5 million bond issue.

"It was kind of a pioneering thing as far as this community was concerned," Wickens remarked. LCH was one of the first hospitals nationwide to practice open staffing and, according to Dr. Denis Radefeld, it was all to the good; the younger D. O.s had backgrounds similar to that of the average M. D., and "they integrated into the staff very easily. The present-day osteopathic surgeon has the equivalent training."

There was also the general resistance to the idea of a second

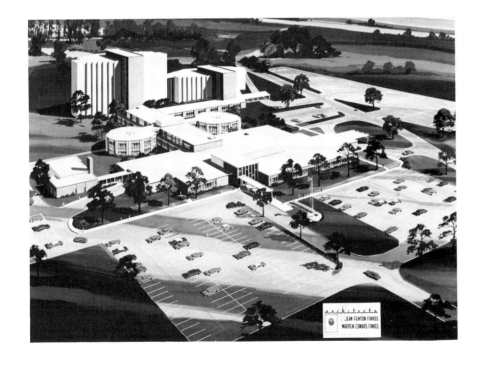

Architects Jean and Warren Finkel's vision for the new hospital featured two circular wings with tall towers. The circular wings were a new concept in hospital design. With a nurses' station at the center of the circle, nurses were no more than just a few steps away from any patient.

TRUE PUBLIC SPIRIT

Seventeen business and industrial concerns, one civic organization, and one individual in the Lorain area helped provide initial operating funds for the new Lorain Community Hospital, which opened its doors to patients May 18, 1964, according to Edward Mehrer, then President of the hospital Board of Trustees. "The civic-minded group will serve as guarantors in underwriting $145,000 needed to pay expenses for operating the hospital until money received for services begins to come in," he said. "Without such a guarantee of funds, our operations would have been impossible, and our board, as well as the community at large, is deeply grateful to this group," Mehrer declared.

Guarantors include:
The American Ship Building Co.
American Crucible Products Co.
Bob Beck Chevrolet
Bettcher Industries of Vermilion
S. W. Becker Motors
Cleveland Electric
Illuminating Co.
Ford Motor Co. Fund
Fruehauf Trailer Co.
Gregory Industries, Inc.
The Lorain Journal
Lorain Products Co.
Lorain Telephone Co.
M. O'Neil Co.
J. C. Penney Co.
Viking Steel Co. of Cleveland
Wakefield Foundation
of Vermilion
Work Wear Co. of Cleveland

The individual mentioned as one of the guarantors was Miss Grace Standen; the civic organization was the Civic and Community Affairs Department of the Lakeland Woman's Club.

From The Lorain Journal,
May 2, 1964

hospital, but the actual need at that time for additional hospital beds was inescapable. A speaker's bureau sent representatives to any group that would listen to their reasons for building the new hospital.

Some doubters were won over when local architects Jean and Warren Finkel unveiled their innovative plans for a truly modern hospital. They had designed circular patient units, which allowed nurses to monitor and care for their charges with ease and efficiency from a central hublike location. Other highlights included functional grouping of surgical suites, extra-wide entrances for safety and efficiency, and escalators to ease traffic jams at the elevators.

And politics inevitably entered the picture—the side-taking, *quid pro quo*, compromise kind of dealing that is the backbone of American life. Once the decision had been made to seek funds through a bond issue, city government became an active player in the game of building the hospital. Technicalities, rules, and precedents had to be respected, and the new hospital had to become a legal entity.

A municipality had the right to build a hospital. It could float bonds to pay for a hospital. But Lorain was hesitant to take on the expense and administration of such a facility. Everyone knew that the millions needed for construction were only the start; there would be huge, ongoing obligations. They wanted the hospital, but . . .

The Hospital Facilities Committee and the women behind it were willing to continue carrying their burden. Ohio laws allowed the city to lease the hospital to some nonprofit organization. The city had only to appoint a special committee when the bond issue passed, and that committee's job would be to find such an organization and oversee their activities.

The Lakeland Community Hospital, Inc., dba Lorain Community Hospital, came into being on September 16, 1961. Members of the group were T. J. McGeachie, Arthur J. Pelander, Miss Grace Standen, Dr. B. C. Myers, Dr. J. H. Dickason, and attorneys Andrew Warhola and Ray Miraldi.

With the medical-osteopathic problems, public relations problems, and legal problems under control and the ground duly broken with gold-colored shovels, it remained only to build the hospital.

Only one problem remained: money!

There would be income from the second Follies and the other projects that demanded hours of work and devotion from countless volunteers.

A second traditional source of funding for nonprofit causes was often a statutory part of their organization: its Board of Trustees. Boards of Trustees are responsible for setting broad policy and serving as liaison to the community. And, when necessary, they find resources for the organization they govern.

On February 27, 1963, the Lorain Community Hospital Trustees held their first annual meeting in the conference room at the Ford Motor Company. Edward Mehrer was elected President and Paul Friedlander

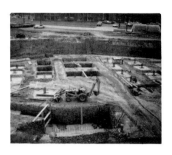

The community watched as the site was cleared for its new hospital at 3700 Kolbe Road on the west side of Lorain.

Vice President. The Board's Secretary was Grace Standen; A. J. Pelander served as Treasurer.

Edward Mehrer was General Manager of the new Ford Motor Company plant in Lorain. He remembered wandering into his office one day, his mind was focused on many difficult problems in the plant, to discover a committee of women waiting for him. Still occupied with the situation he had left moments before, he half-listened to their request. Such a worthy cause! And his company had such a fine record for community support in communities where it had factories! And all they needed was a tiny bit of his time and expertise. . . . He agreed.

He little dreamed that his sincere but absent-minded assent would

The main lobby was spaciously designed, with large windows and individual seating areas for the enjoyment of visitors, 1964.

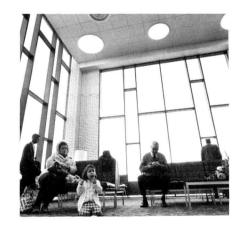

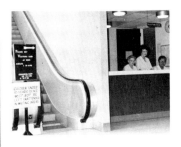

lead to his becoming the first President of Lorain Community Hospital.

As Board President, his first priority was to increase operating funds; the hospital was lacking many basic instruments and such everyday necessities as linens. He persuaded the Ford Motor Company to furnish a 180-degree x-ray table; later, when needs expanded, he arranged for an upgrade to a 360-degree table.

Part of the Board's job was to importune additional funds from the City Council. In February, 1964, the city agreed to a plea for $40,000 for additional equipment. Two months later, they approved an expenditure of $25,000 for improved water lines on Kolbe Road; they had once again been won over and made to appreciate the importance of fire protection to the future patients of LCH.

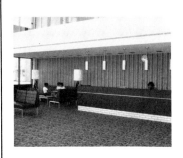

Mehrer was also responsible for recruiting an administrator. After a year-long search, James E. Huson of Parkersburg, West Virginia, was hired on November 1, 1963.

Ford transferred Mehrer in 1964, and Charles Herzer took temporary leadership of the Board. A grateful community was pleased to place Mehrer's portrait in the lobby of the hospital he had done so much to promote. The executive claimed that seeing his picture hung in that impressive entryway was a great moment.

"I guess it made me prouder than anything I've done in my life."

But before the lobby existed, the building had to go up. Bulldozers like the one June Steen had driven at the ground-breaking ceremony were

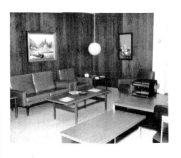

Escalators took visitors from the lobby to the patient level of the hospital.

Photographed in May, 1964, the lobby was decorated with very modern wall and floor coverings. The lobby was first remodeled in 1978.

Considered ultra modern, the executive offices in 1964 were comfortable and efficient.

cranked into high gear. Truckloads of materials arrived; construction workers and craftsmen toiled under the interested eyes of passers-by. The community watched as the hospital grew.

Finally, the moment had arrived. The dream was about to be realized. The journey had progressed to its first destination. And the prophecy of Vernon Siefer of Fairview Hospital in 1957—that the process would take seven years—was fulfilled, almost to the day.

The hospital was dedicated on Sunday, April 30, 1964. Buses had

Jack Snell inspects boiler-room equipment.

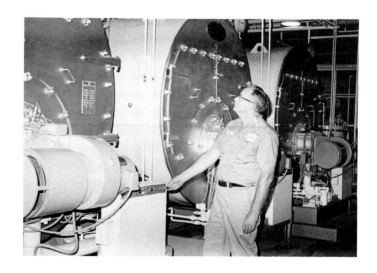

been shuttling excited guests from the loop in downtown since noon. At 1:00 P. M., the Honorable Woodrow Mathna, Mayor of Lorain, made his opening remarks. Together with Leo Svete and Edward Mehrer, he ceremoniously cut the ribbon that officially opened the hospital. There were bands playing, flags flying, prayers and speeches, and even good wishes from the White House.

The open house treated visitors to glimpses of the new hospital not usually on view. They could tour the three operating rooms, two delivery

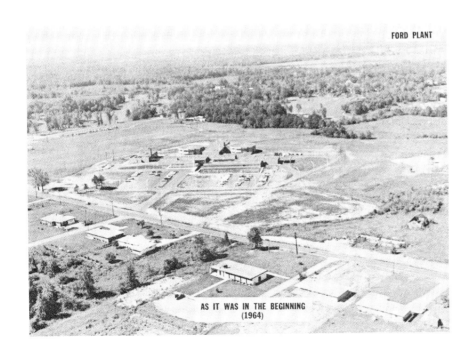

Lorain Community Hospital, 1964. With 150 beds, it was the third largest hospital in the County.

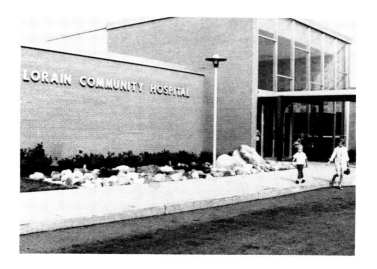

The new hospital opened in May, 1964 and featured two major operating rooms, one minor operating room, a cystoscopic room and two delivery rooms.

rooms (subsequently not opened in the interest of consolidating and not adding a third obstetrics hospital to the Lorain area), and a cystoscopic room, where exploratory x-rays would be taken and developed. They could visit the pair of pharmacies, one each for outpatients and resident patients. They could exclaim over the pleasant rooms for patients, the serene chapel, the spacious lobby, and the efficient-looking offices.

Everything was bright and new and clean, and cries of "How nice!" and "How lovely!" could be heard as guests discovered additional features.

Mingling with the visitors at the dedication were many who would serve the hospital. They were looking beyond the party atmosphere to the real "opening day" when patients would begin to arrive. Though the idea of a hospital brings a vision of experienced, knowledgeable doctors and

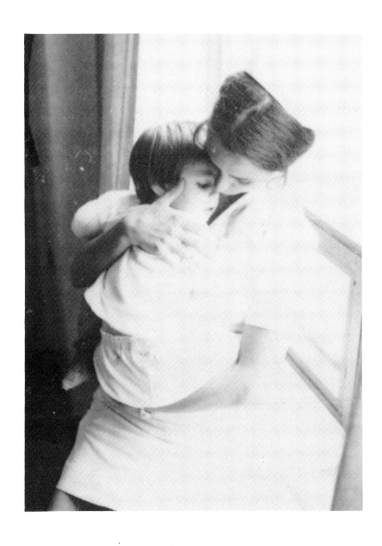

Patients of all ages receive more than medical care. Lorain Community Hospital is where you would want your loved ones should hospitalization be necessary.

efficient, skilled nurses, these people are only one part of the vast team of trained workers necessary to keep a hospital on course.

Under the coordination of Administrator James E. Huson, the new facility could boast ten departments; each would be functioning, if only on a limited basis, when the hospital opened.

Largest of these departments, the nursing service under the direction of Jean Damon, R. N., would be responsible for operating rooms and delivery rooms, nurseries, and patient areas. Eventually, the hospital planned to hire over one hundred nurses, nurse supervisors, aides, and

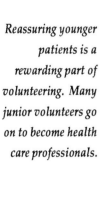

Reassuring younger patients is a rewarding part of volunteering. Many junior volunteers go on to become health care professionals.

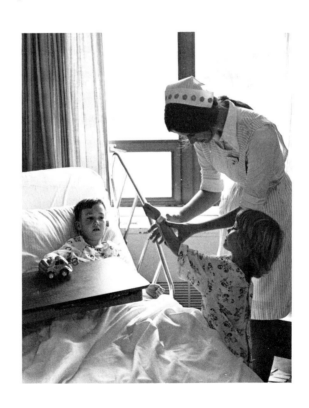

orderlies.

Initially staffed by hospital personnel, the pharmacy would in time become an independent department with its own staff.

Behind the scenes, trained technicians would be stationed in the medical records, x-ray, and laboratory departments. The years after World War II had seen remarkable advances in diagnostic procedures and examination methods. These departments could count on continually upgrading their training and equipment.

Patients, staff, and visitors would be constantly aware of the efforts of the housekeeping department, as porters, maids, and linen service

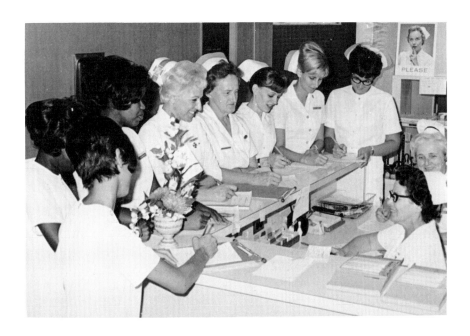

The staff receive their instructions from the shift supervisor.

workers, under the housekeeper's supervision, kept the hospital as spotless as it was at its dedication. They would also notice the work of the dietary department, which kept a score of food service specialists busy preparing special diets for patients as well as providing a cafeteria for staff and visitors.

The plant engineer, with his staff of carpenters and mechanics, would keep the building functioning inside and out, and the purchasing department would see that the storerooms were supplied with the "million-and-one" items needed by each area.

The switchboard, admitting office, information desk, and financial areas such as billing, bookkeeping, and the cashier's office, would be the province of the business department.

Among the guests of honor at the dedication were the members of the city's Hospital Facilities Commission. They had reason to congratulate themselves; they had overseen every aspect of the hospital's existence since the passage of the bond issue. The four original members, Ruth Calta, Steve Szuhy, Leo Svete, and Lewis Goodell and ex officio member Mayor Woodrow Mathna did not regret the Commission's imminent demise; its original work was completed with the construction of the building. Its future role for many years would be to oversee subsequent changes of the facility. They knew the undertaking was far from finished; as individuals they would continue supporting Lorain Community Hospital in countless other ways.

CHAPTER THREE

A Perilous Infancy:
The First Three Years

There is a maxim in the Midwest that concerns spending your last dime for a purse to put it in. Unkind observers might have sat back and waited for Lorain Community Hospital, in its shiny newness, to wither away for lack of additional funding.

The first patient, Mrs. Frank Trepoy, was admitted on May 25, 1964. She was lavished with care during her historic stay. Even when the novelty wore off, the quality of care did not diminish, as more pioneer patients were admitted to the twenty-bed medical unit originally in use. It had been decided to open gradually; easing into the complex health care undertaking seemed prudent. Surgical cases would be accepted by the beginning of June. Emergency room staffing, a house physician, and interns would follow in time.

By August of that year, the hospital had served 458 patients; the average stay was seven-plus days. By year's end over 1,500 patients had been treated, about half medical and half surgical. There were eighty doctors on staff and over one hundred other personnel.

The earliest patients were attended by practitioners under the guidance of R. P. Hardwig, M. D., the first Chief of the Medical Staff.

Robert Schmidt was LCH's first chief pharmacist

Stock room supervisor Mike Misita checks inventory of the many necessities for running a hospital.

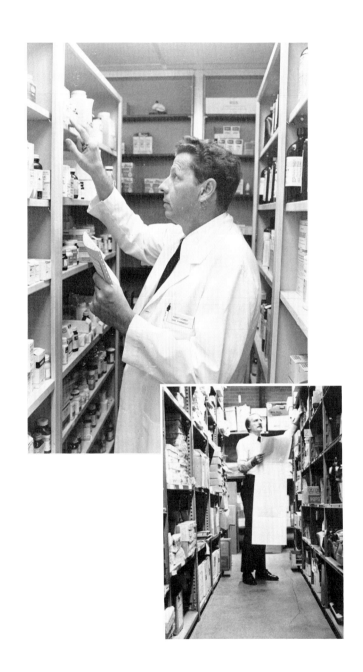

FIRST BIRTH

The first birth at Lorain Community Hospital has already happened! Soon after the building was under construction, a robin built a nest in one of the girders and in, of all places, the part destined to be the maternity wing. She had triplets.

The Lorain Journal,
May 2, 1964

Besides overseeing the interesting novelty of medical doctors working side-by-side with doctors of osteopathy, Dr. Hardwig served as the indispensable link between the Board of Trustees, the medical staff, and the Administration. Good communications were vital, especially when income was almost nonexistent and even a minor detail could easily escalate into a financial crisis.

The first few years were difficult. According to Laurie Hoke, they were "absolutely terrible. We would walk down the street and duck into doorways to avoid our creditors."

These grim memories were triggered by the fact that neither the City of Lorain nor the Lakeland Hospital corporation had any money. "We were on a very limited budget," she recalled, to the depressing point where guarantors were eventually advised that their credit guarantees were actually loans and would eventually be considered gifts. Most of the big-hearted businesses eventually agreed to consider the money as donations to the hospital.

There were ways to survive when money was short. David Ross, then a Board member, recalled:

"We borrowed money from our suppliers by a very simple method: you don't pay your bills. The suppliers were good to us," he added. They shared an underlying conviction that the hospital would survive the hard times and grow; that belief allowed creditors to be patient.

Stanley Pijor, Lorain banker, has long kept a finger on the financial pulse of the hospital. He admits he didn't follow the construction of the hospital too closely and was a bit surprised when he was approached to be its treasurer.

"I figured a hospital of $3 million being built should have adequate working capital, right? I assumed that and accepted the position." On becoming Treasurer a year after the building was completed, Pijor discovered the hospital had a grand total of about $35,000.

"It was a very hard, struggling period of time, those first three years: a lack of working capital, working with suppliers and creditors. Everybody was very understanding; we got extended terms." The creditors were eventually paid off, Pijor recalled, but "over a longer period of time."

Alice Weston's original history repeated a common theme at this point in the hospital's story.

"The women again took on the task. They went to businesses and individuals, asking for loans of $5,000 or more. They raised enough to put the hospital on a sound footing. Many 'ate up the loans' and did not ask for repayment."

Women's groups turned to a nationally advertised money-raising scheme. Under the leadership of Elizabeth King and Jessie Greenwood, volunteers collected Betty Crocker coupons. Thousands were clipped from flour bags and cake-mix boxes by housewives all over the county. When their envelopes and bundles of coupons were tallied, Lorain's effort

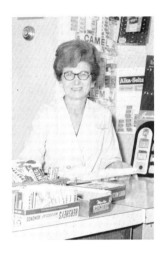

won—over many larger cities. The award money went to purchase the hospital's first telemeter. Such a basic piece of equipment, used to measure vital body signs, was gratefully accepted by the hospital; over the years, the number of telemeters in use grew many times over.

Physicians, frequently more aware than anyone of gaps in apparatus inventories, often provided funds for needed equipment for their own work.

Many city and county organizations, unions, fraternal groups, and clubs gave money for needed items. But it was women's groups, such as the Steel City Grandmothers, that exerted themselves especially to help "the hospital the women built."

"It is amazing how a hospital came along with no money and a lot of guts," David Ross observed.

The hospital suffered a substantial setback when the Ford Motor Company transferred Edward Mehrer from Lorain in late 1964. Institutions should be more than a sum of their members, but individuals have a way of seeming indispensable.

Long-time hospital supporter and Board member Charles Herzer stepped in as interim President, but his business responsibilities made the level of dedication he felt the hospital deserved impossible. Paul Friedlander, Assistant General Manager of U. S. Steel, then assumed the presidency.

Though Charles Herzer served only a short time as President of the

During the early days of the Treasure Chest, Marie Wilson, the Tuesday Chairman of Volunteers, greets patrons with a welcoming smile.

Board, his successor praised him for his contributions in those early years. "Charles Herzer was one of the finest men I have ever known and a great asset to the Board."

Friedlander, who served as President of the Board of Trustees from 1965 to 1974, also honored the efforts of labor union executive Clyde Jackson. Each Board member did yeoman duty during the difficult early years. They worked quietly and efficiently and usually admitted that their best efforts were matched by the dedicated women of Lorain who were so instrumental in founding the hospital.

One of the Board's early acts both honored and institutionalized the efforts of the women who were so dedicated to the hospital. In

The Treasure Chest is operated for the benefit of the hospital by the LCH Auxiliary. Volunteer Jennie Bresak inspects one of the store's "treasures."

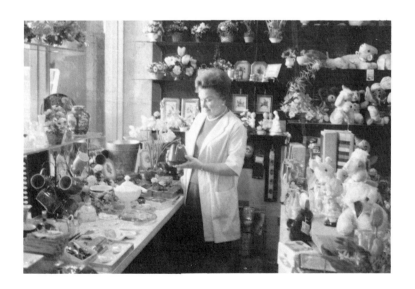

November, 1964 the Trustees urged the women to form an auxiliary. An autonomous organization dedicated to its interests, "womaned" with proven "movers and shakers," would be a boon to the new hospital. Mrs. George Hoke (who would serve as the Auxiliary's first president), Mrs. Elmer Steen, and Miss Grace Standen were formally appointed by the Board to get the Auxiliary started.

If ever an organization was inevitable, the Lorain Community Hospital Auxiliary was that group. The first meeting attracted 150 potential members! By December, the numbers had swelled to 300 members, representing fifty-two women's organizations.

From the beginning, the Auxiliary was a true community activity. All were welcome who were willing to contribute fifty hours a year to the hospital's needs. The group was even proud to admit several bold-spirited males into their fold.

There was no letup in fund-raising activities once the Auxiliary was operating, but a second, equally important facet of the group's activities was organized—volunteering. Ruth Calta was the first volunteer chair.

Volunteers, like love, "make the world go round," and they served a vital part in the life of Lorain Community Hospital. Many of the faces a visitor or patient remembered most from a hospital visit were those of volunteers. At the information desks, in offices and halls, hard-working volunteers could be found. They visited lonely patients; they delivered the mail. They dispensed coffee, library books, information, and understanding with friendly smiles. Some were young; teenagers, students, and young mothers brightened the halls with their enthusiasm and good nature. Some were merely young at heart: helping in the hospital was the perfect job for retired people too spirited to be idle.

On St. Patrick's Day, 1965, the hospital's gift shop, the Treasure Chest, opened its doors. Besides providing small comforts and necessities to patients and guests, the gift shop's profits helped plump the hospital's always slim purse.

The limited number of beds available when the hospital first opened its doors soon grew. As each twenty-bed unit opened, it became

Jean Hunker, chair of the teen volunteers, helps distribute floral arrangements.

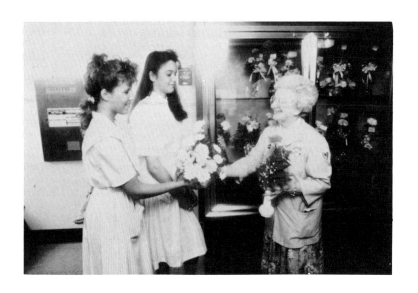

36

busy with the rustle of starched skirts, the calm announcements of intercoms, the whirr of equipment strange to visitor eyes. By March, 1965, less than a year after dedication, 94 of 150 hospital beds had opened. The Board discussed the need for additional parking; could they ask the city for $3,000 to cover the curbs and street access?

There were, in fact, more patients than the nurses could care for. Among the changes that developed in the sixties was a substantial drop in the number of registered nurses available to work in an increasing number of hospitals across the nation. Other doors were beginning to open for women who wanted careers. The arduous years of training were not so appealing as they had been when nursing was one of the few opportunities open to women. An article in *The Lorain Journal* announced:

"Today, that magnificent medical edifice Lorain Community Hospital is going begging . . . begging for registered nurses!" The article sent out a plea to former nurses to come out of retirement, if only for a year, for the community good. The appeal went beyond the city limits as well. In its recruiting attempts, the Administration attracted three nurses from faraway Scotland.

Eventually, LCH, possibly due to what *The Lorain Journal* described as "everything possible for splendid working conditions," was able to hire adequate staff. By the following year, a Candy Striper Program was instituted. Young girls, clad in cheerful pink-and-white pinafores, worked with nurses and other staff; it was hoped that the teen-aged volunteers

Lorain Community Hospital's success can be attributed to the hard work of many individuals.

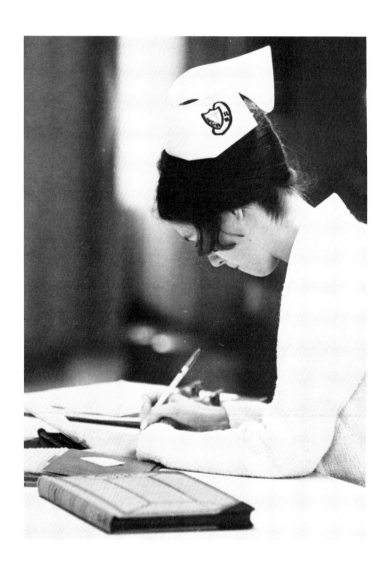

would eventually consider hospital careers.

Alice Weston's original chronicles marked a high point in 1967, three years after the hospital's dedication. Before plans for the osteopathic hospital, Lorain General, had been shelved, supporters had collected money for that cause. The funds had been quietly gathering interest for years. Since doctors of osteopathy were welcome at Lorain Community Hospital, a court order directed the money to be divided between LCH and Amherst Hospital, where D. O.s also practiced. The fund at that time totaled $50,190.15.

"When your bills get extended to as much as a year to eighteen months, you know you have major problems," banker Stan Pijor observed. "But when you get your bills down to a thirty- to forty-five-day basis, then you are in a comfortable working capital position."

They had made it through a truly perilous part of the journey. Bills were paid, payrolls met, suppliers cheerfully offering credit. There were hopeful patients being admitted every day, and satisfied patients going home. The dream—and the journey—would continue.

*Karen Shullick comforts
the emergency care
center's first patient,
April 3, 1972.*

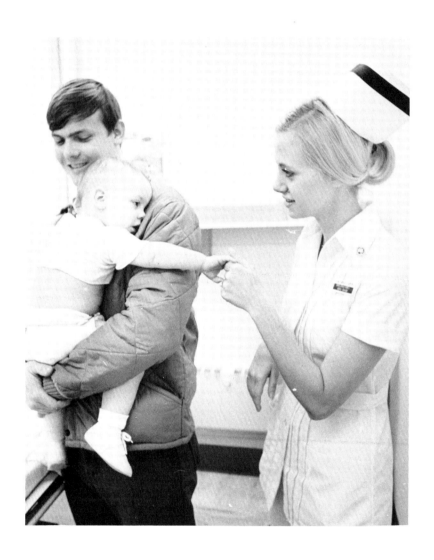

CHAPTER FOUR

A Promising Childhood: Completing the First Decade

Once the crushing worry of finance was eased, the hospital was able to better respond to the needs of the community. Without agonized concern about daily expenses, it was possible to move on to the next part of the journey. It was possible to grow.

The original twenty-bed capacity had, of course, quickly expanded, and by 1966, the original 150-bed plan had been realized. The hospital had been designed with such flexibility that it was possible to add extra beds in areas designed for other purposes.

Fifteen beds were added to the count when it was decided that Lorain Community Hospital did not need an obstetrics department. The birthrate was down; St. Joseph and Amherst hospitals could easily handle obstetric services in the Lorain area. The maternity ward was converted into much-needed general-purpose rooms, and the bed-count of the hospital surpassed its original expectations. LCH had patients waiting for every medical-surgical bed that could be fit into its rooms; sometimes there was even an overflow into corridors. Generous use of health care resources was growing at an accelerated rate across the country, and public expectations in Lorain were equally great.

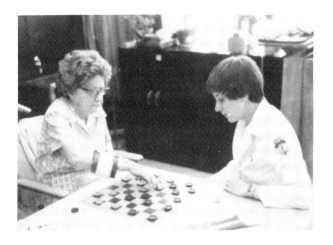

Physical therapy, though sometimes fun and games, returns independence to patients who have suffered from strokes, accidents, and other illnesses.

It was time to think big. Consultant Ross Garrett was asked to help with the hospital's plans for the future.

Paul Friedlander, President of the Board of Trustees, was forced to resign when his company transferred him to Pittsburgh. Another member of the Board, David Ross, who had been head of the planning committee, was asked to become the new Board President.

"I probably had the most exciting job at the hospital, developing new approaches," David Ross told historian Alice Weston. "The community was unified through the efforts of Ross Garrett. Ross [Garret] had vision that the proper-sized hospital should really be tailored to meet the demands of the patients specifically. He recognized and developed an approach where intensity of service was available to those who were extremely ill, less extremely ill, and those with relatively minor problems."

While long-range planning continued, new services for the people of Lorain were presented as soon as they could be implemented. In the fall of 1967, a physical therapy section was opened, complete with two treatment rooms—$3,000 worth of therapy equipment and a full-time therapist, Patrick L. Cozzie. Physical therapy was an area in which Candy Stripers and hospital volunteers made a large difference. Under the supervision of Dr. Maynard Brucker, they worked many hours to help sore and diseased limbs to function again.

In response to a serious community need, the first alcohol detoxification center was started in the main building. Though it started small, this program was destined to be one of the most noteworthy at LCH.

Four years after the hospital first opened, a major expansion program was unveiled.

"A $3.5 million expansion program at Lorain Community Hospital was approved by the hospital Board of Trustees last night," *The Lorain Journal* reported on May 29, 1968. Ross Garrett announced a long-term plan that included a ten-story structure of one-patient rooms and a five-story building for convalescent patients. Phase I would include the basement and three stories of the taller structure, which would rise west of the existing facility. Building should start within one year, he promised, with completion eighteen months after construction started.

Paul Friedlander pointed out that the present building was designed "in a manner to permit economical expansion." He added that the "question is no longer are we needed but, rather, how can we keep up with the needs of this dramatically growing community and its medical service expectations?" Population had grown by almost 10,000 in ten years; the 1970 census registered 78,185. Those needs included a coronary-care unit, full-time pathology service, and expanded clinical laboratory services.

Another $3.5 million? It seemed only yesterday that citizens had

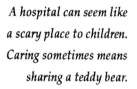

A hospital can seem like a scary place to children. Caring sometimes means sharing a teddy bear.

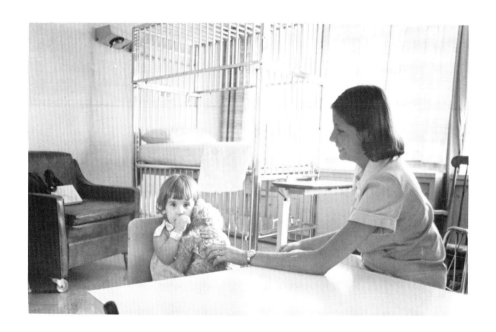

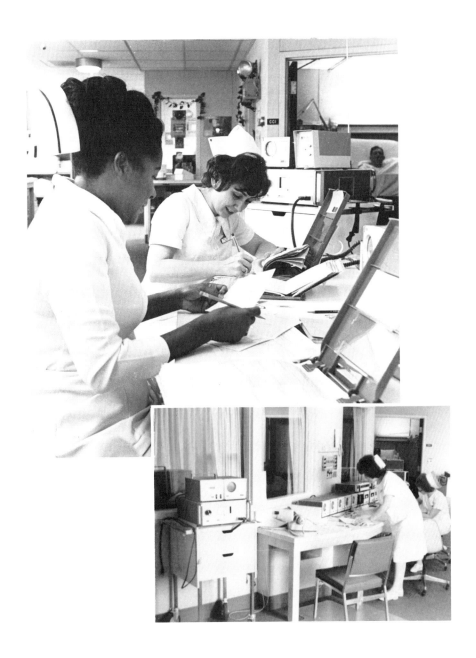

The new hospital was designed so that nurses could keep a close vigil on patients. Studies have shown that patients are more relaxed when nurses are within view.

Nurses working in the coronary care unit in 1970

had that figure buzzing in their ears when the original building was still an elaborate dream. It had been a good investment, that bond issue. Passing another bond issue to enlarge LCH would not be the life-or-death crisis its supporters had lived through in 1960. And in the long run, it would be much less painful than a public subscription drive. It would be a good investment; the voters had been assured of that. The bond issue of 1968 passed.

James Huson left as Administrator in the spring of 1968; the hospital functioned under acting executive director Ross Garrett.

The interim administration ran the hospital while conducting a search for a permanent director. Recommended by Ross Garrett, George O. West was appointed to the post in the late autumn of 1968. He found a facility operating in the black, its staff capable and content, its long-range planning ambitious. Architects Finkel and Finkel were preparing blueprints that would enlarge the medical facility to triple its present size.

In 1971, four floors of the tower were finished, housing a young-adult center, a detoxification unit for alcoholics, a psychiatric center, and a children's ward. A fifth floor was shelled in. The structure was built to support seven floors if needed.

More celebration attended the opening of the Emergency Care Center in April, 1972.

"Over 400 people participated in the ribbon cutting ceremony," Alice Weston reported. "The excitement of providing this much-needed service was expressed by all in attendance, especially the emergency and rescue unit personnel from Lorain and neighboring communities.

"The emergency care facility added a new dimension of health care service, and one month later a [Regional] Poison Control Center was established to address another medical care need for the community—the first in the county."

In 1973, the completed diamond shaped tower addition was opened. The hospital's new cardiac treatment center was considered one of the best in the area. There was even a helicopter landing pad at the door of the emergency room.

As always, the Auxiliary was busy, continuing both its volunteer work and its fund-raising with what seemed to be an unending supply of enthusiasm.

Their comprehensive scrapbook held a collection of editorial clips that would make any group beam with pride. "The entire community owes the LCH Auxiliary a resounding vote of thanks." (5-27-66) "There's a word for it: ASTOUNDING. That is the [exclamation] which comes forth when the activities of the Lorain Community Hospital Auxiliary are described." (11-12-66)

When Auxiliary President June Steen gave $10,000 from the Auxiliary toward a new fund in May, 1968, it raised to $85,975 the amount contributed since the hospital opened. A half-dozen years later, the total had risen to $315,000.

ACCREDITATION

On February 19, 1969, the hospital received full accreditation from the Joint Commission on Accreditation of Hospitals for a term of three years.

The Joint Commission was formed in 1951. It is a nonprofit, nongovernmental organization currently sponsored by four major hospital and medical organizations —the American College of Physicians, the American College of Surgeons, the American Hospital Association, the American Medical Association.

Since 1969, Lorain Community Hospital has continued full accreditation.

In late 1974, *The Lorain Journal* reported: "Two years ago the organization set a new goal, and pledged that it would earn a quarter of a million dollars for the hospital in three years. With this week's gift of $87,778, they have already reached $244,000, only $6,000 short of the goal." Eight months ahead of schedule, in December, 1974, they reached their $250,000 objective.

At their tenth anniversary celebration, the volunteers honored their

Aerial of Lorain
Community Hospital in
1973

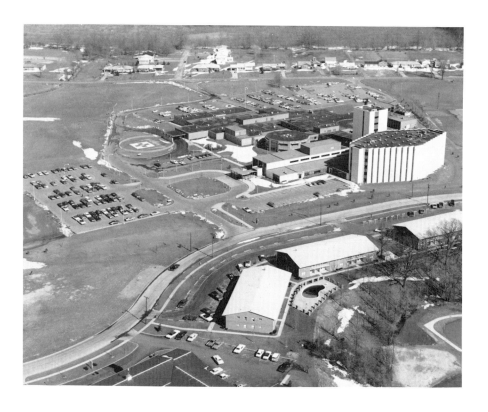

members' contribution of more than 47,000 hours of service that year, plus another 11,000 hours from the Candy Stripers. "For the first time, the Auxiliary felt it was fluent enough to afford a token gift; they weren't required to buy their tickets to the affair," the paper reported. Over ten years, they had provided $518,355.04.

In addition to the liberality of the Auxiliary in contributing to the hospital's income, two generous women had provided bequests that continued to aid the facility through the years.

Grace Standen, longtime supporter of LCH, died in 1970. In an era that offered few career opportunities to women, at the age of twenty-eight, Miss Standen had decided to make finance her life's work. Before the outbreak of World War I, she joined the National Bank of Commerce (now Lorain National Bank), moving to their trust department three years later. She became a trust officer for the National Bank of Lorain in 1935, and rose to vice president and director of that bank by the end of World War II. For years Secretary of the hospital's Board of Trustees, she established a trust "for the purchase and acquisition of medical, surgical and hospital equipment for Lorain Community Hospital." Her bequest to the hospital provided thousands of dollars a year for needed materials and equipment.

Grace Standen was not the only open-handed woman to endow the hospital. Gladys Hills Irish, a Lorain native whose family was associated with the Lorain National Bank, started a trust for the hospital while she was still living, designed to "be invested for the use and benefit of Lorain Community Hospital . . . in purchasing supplies and equipment for said hospital, in making contributions toward operation of said hospital." The hospital has received earnings from the trust yearly; in early 1974, they were given a check for over $11,000.

By its tenth year, the value of the hospital's assets had exceeded $17 million.

But a hospital is more than bricks and mortar, even more than the devoted work of volunteers and the loyalty of patients and well-wishers. One of the most vital elements of a healing institution is the integrity and standards of its medical staff. In an era fraught with challenges for the medical calling, Lorain's doctors worked hard to keep their ethical and professional criteria high. From the earliest days, they had the backing of the whole institution.

"The sense of cooperation among the Administration, the Board of Trustees, and medical staff has not changed but has continued to grow abundantly," said Dr. Denis Radefeld, one of the original LCH doctors and former Chief of Staff. "I have never seen a place where a Board of Trustees has been more interested in what is going on. There may have been a reasonable level of involvement—up until we had a major physician-related crisis. Specifically we had to throw one physician off the staff, and he sued."

The situation, which eventually involved elements that could grace the most bizarre of horror novels, caused considerable publicity and embarrassment to the hospital. The Board and Administration, however, were impeccable in their united support for the medical staff's actions.

"The hospital became recognized as an institution that had guts enough to throw somebody off their staff, if there was somebody who they felt wasn't performing appropriately," Dr. Radefeld continued. "There were three other physicians who were dismissed from the staff because of incompetency; they didn't live up to a standard. They were expected to perform from 'excellent' to a level that is still acceptable. If they fell below that line they had to go back for additional training." The three doctors, he added, returned to practice after completing the required instruction.

Dedicated to the highest possible standards, the medical staff

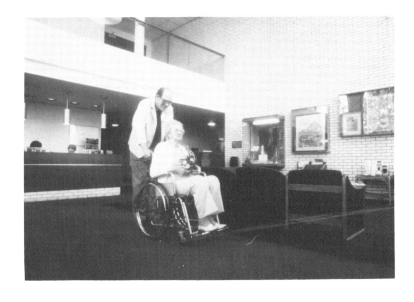

People volunteer for many different reasons, some to gain experience for future careers in medicine, others to contribute to society. Volunteers continue their commitment to serving others at Lorain Community Hospital.

submits to rigorous review committees who oversee their work. Dr. Radefeld commented that "the success of these efforts is reflected in the fact that LCH has one of the better malpractice records among those covered by their insurance company."

"A decade of progress in the medical world was celebrated last night as administrators, medical staff, volunteers and friends attended the Tenth Annual Report Dinner of the Lorain Community Hospital," *The Lorain Journal* reported on May 1, 1974. Among the guests of honor was Edward Mehrer, who traveled from his home in Canada for the event. He shared a table with Paul Friedlander, who had recently announced that his company, U.S. Steel, had transferred him to Pittsburgh. The Board would

Four friendly volunteers working the Treasure Chest (left to right): Marie Wilson, Fritz Gerber, Arlene Gerber, and Valeska Cuthbert.

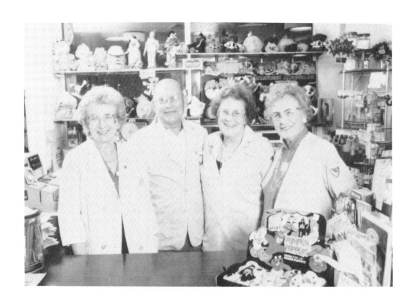

soon need to choose itself a new president.

Four months after the tenth anniversary celebration, George West resigned as Administrator; he planned to direct a retirement center in Florida. Harold Bregman, Trustee, became the Acting Administrator, supported by the expertise of consultant Ross Garrett. Bregman interrupted his retirement to help the hospital; according to David Ross, he "was willing to do any job—and he was a top-notch executive."

"He had the interest and the time and the dedication," Laurie Hoke remembered. "He did a wonderful job."

Moving into a second decade, the Board once again cast its net, seeking the best possible leadership for the hospital.

The Great Lakes Regional Rehabilitation Center assists in restoring patients to the highest practical level of self-sufficiency. Each patient has a program designed specifically for his or her needs. Becky McClain, P T Assistant III, works with a patient.

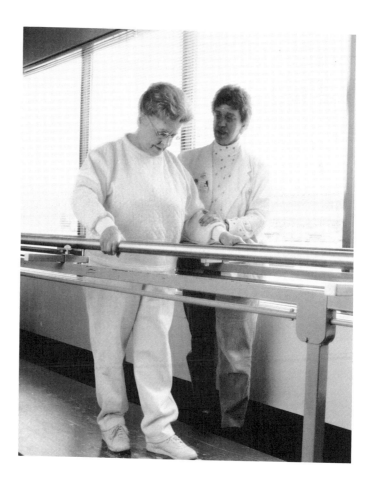

CHAPTER FIVE

Better and Better: Leadership in the Growing Years

Lorain Community Hospital faced the next leg of its journey from a fairly high plateau. While there had been challenges, they had been met. If there were rough places in the road ahead, there was also confidence that the journey would go on.

The loss of Board President Paul Friedlander was a considerable one; until U. S. Steel transferred him to Pittsburgh, his years of leadership had been an important part of the hospital's success. The post was assumed by long-time Board member David Ross, who had the advantage of association with a local company: no untimely transfers were likely. Ross was an assertive and indefatigable advocate of the hospital; sometimes provoking controversy, he was willing to cross swords, if necessary, for the good of the organization. He served from 1974 until 1984.

One of the first tasks for the Board was to recruit the best possible executive director for the hospital. Laurie Hoke remembered that each director, in his turn, had made a contribution: "They were all wonderful. The right man was here at the right moment."

Mr. and Mrs. Paul Balcom were welcomed to Lorain Community Hospital at an introductory tea. Steve Speckhart from the maintenance department introduces himself to the new Executive Director.

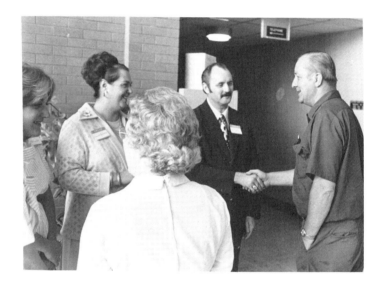

In March, 1975, Paul Balcom was selected to be the hospital's new Executive Director. He came to the position with a strong background in both medical and administrative areas. He had a reputation as a "consulting doctor for ailing hospitals," according to an article in *The Lorain Journal.* "Lorain Community Hospital isn't sick in the least," the paper pointed out. "Why is he here?" The problems facing the Lorain hospital hardly compared to previous positions where Balcom had struggled with convoluted financial predicaments, horrendous morale problems, and decayed community relations. The answer concerned priorities and lifestyles. As Corporate Vice President and Regional Director for a major national hospital management company, Balcom had found he was spending more and more time traveling and less and less time with his family. Despite challenges and fulfillments associated with multihospital management responsibilities, his preference was to focus on a single hospital directorship. Lorain Community Hospital, he told *The Lorain Journal* "is a first-class hospital both in physical plant and potential. The potential is fantastic." In addition, the location was appealing. His wife, Claire, had relatives in nearby Cleveland, and the Balcom children, Steven, Pamela, and Karen, would benefit from Lorain's excellent school system.

Balcom's choice of vocation was in part directed by a cousin who, as a psychiatrist and hospital administrator, introduced him to the fascinating complexity of the modern hospital. As a practitioner, this mentor was aware of the gap between management skills and healing arts and pointed out that a good hospital administrator should have a solid background in both fields. With a bachelor's degree in nursing, a master's degree in hospital administration, and an administrative residency at the John Hopkins Hospital, Balcom had spent twenty years in hospital management before being chosen to direct Lorain Community Hospital.

When he started in his new position in June, 1975, Paul Balcom made clear to the Board that he wanted to run a facility with reasonable rates and costs comparable to other area hospitals, but that it was important to maintain a profit margin of 5 percent of the net revenue. Without that kind of solid financial base, he pointed out, a hospital cannot grow in either clinical excellence or program diversification. And growth was as vital to a hospital as to any concern. He agreed with banker Stan Pijor that "you really have to start running a hospital like any other business. I think it is healthy in the long run."

The plans for growth that he outlined were exciting and

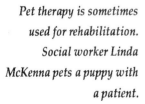

Pet therapy is sometimes used for rehabilitation. Social worker Linda McKenna pets a puppy with a patient.

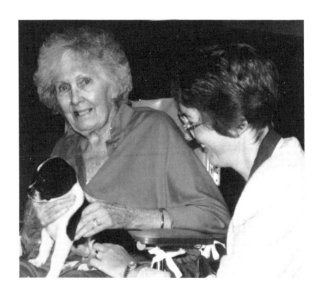

Better and Better:
Leadership in the Growing Years

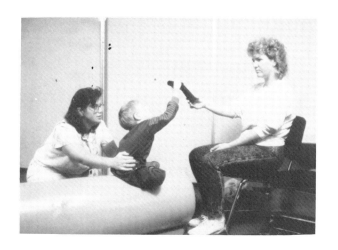

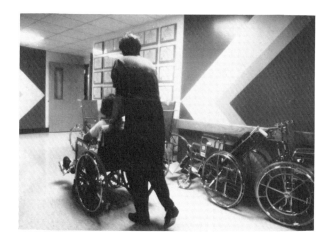

Occupational therapy is not necessarily therapy dealing with one's occupation. It helps individuals improve the skills they need for everyday life. Christopher Kaya and his mother work with occupational therapist Carol Fischer.

Arrows on the walls and carpet point the way for visitors to find their desired destination.

demonstrated the most progressive concepts in health care. Ideas like meals-on-wheels, checkups for diabetics, and other preventive medicine programs seemed at first self-defeating. They were designed to keep people out of hospitals! But in reality, the end product of a successful hospital is a healthy community. The sick, like the poor, we always have with us. A socially responsible organization like Lorain Community Hospital must be committed to caring for the medical needs of the poor and near-poor as well as those economically advantaged.

Unfortunately, the painful facts of economic life force some of these desirable programs into lower priorities in the overall health care picture.

Even small improvements in muscle strength can make a difference in the life of a patient recovering from accident or illness. Brenda Ely, P T Assistant III, encourages patients with her enthusiasm.

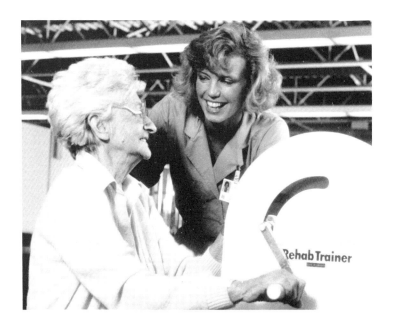

Better and Better:
Leadership in the Growing Years

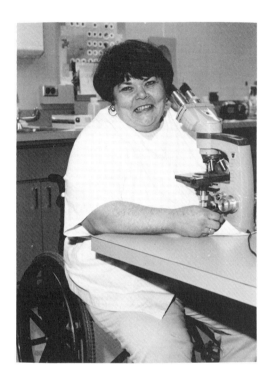

After 13 years of employment at LCH, Mary Susan Grieve experienced the Rehabilitation Program first hand. Since her accident, she has been confined to a wheelchair but continues to be a highly productive and dedicated employee. The experience with Mary Susan Grieve exemplifies Lorain Community Hospital's commitment to accommodate the needs of physically limited employees who can significantly contribute to the institutional mission.

But programs that educate, that prevent disease, mean better use of resources for the more severe cases. Humane and effective treatment can also be cost-effective. Another approach to growth was the constant improvement of the quality of medical care. As older physicians retired, it was vital to attract the most talented and skilled replacements. Excellent doctors were interviewed from top-notch hospitals all over the United States and in many foreign countries. There was also a special effort to recruit from nearer home. If local people, completing their medical education at the nation's finest establishments, chose Lorain Community Hospital over a worldwide pick of assignments, it was a special triumph and a compliment to both hospital and community. This focused physician-recruitment effort was highly successful in "bringing home" many of greater Lorain's finest young citizens.

Though family practice remained important, many new medical specialties were developing during the sixties and seventies. LCH saw the value of offering a location for these innovative techniques to flourish. An example was the hospital's response to the need for a special unit for ophthalmology and the subsequent development of a major Eye Referral Center. New approaches to diseases of the eye were being discovered. Lorain County's first corneal transplant, for example, was performed at LCH's new center by Dr. John Costin. Innovative doctors and new techniques required up-to-date equipment and highly skilled support associates. Technology made great strides in almost every field, and the results, in both diagnosis and treatment, seemed nearly miraculous.

This form of expansion was, however, very expensive. James L. Bardoner, Lorain businessman, originally joined the Board in 1975. One of his initial Board duties concerned approving a $350,000 purchase of esoteric but necessary equipment and required assurances from the administration and physicians that the purchase would be essential to quality patient care and financially justified.

Paying the bills was, in general, an unglamorous business, and the same big-hearted people continued to accept the burden. With commendable promptness, the Auxiliary presented hard-earned checks to the Board, the fruits of endless hours of work in the hospital's gift shop and snack bar, as well as events like the spring "Nearly New Sale." A continuing "big ticket" event was the Follies, which took on a patriotic theme in the Bicentennial year. The paper's headline, "Local big shots put aside dignity for good cause," summed up the generous and unstuffy spirit of business executives, social leaders, and political figures willing to help the hospital. The 1976 financial report presented to Lorain citizens by its hospital seemed to exemplify the progress-through-cooperation theme of the nation's 200th birthday.

Looking back to the original twenty-bed operation, Stan Pijor reported that the hospital's growth had been remarkable. The original bill of $3.5 million was being reduced and would be completely paid off in 1982; the cost to each taxpayer averaged about four dollars per year. Over a dozen years the hospital had become one of the largest locally owned and managed businesses; with planned expansion, its payroll would top 800 employees.

The expansion undertaken in 1968 had been prudent in more ways than one; not only were the additions worthwhile when they were built, but their good timing allowed LCH to charge the lowest semiprivate bed rate ($106) in the area years later.

As important as dollars and cents might be to the running of the

WINTER OF '77-78

Jack Frost was especially busy the winter of 1977-1978 in the Lorain area. The cold and snowy winter inconvenienced many citizens and caused the hospital Auxiliary to postpone its famous Follies, "due to bad winter weather." Despite the inconvenience, the show eventually provided the hospital with a whopping $19,000 profit. Some of those dollars may have been earmarked for the phone-equipped "bad-weather shelters" included in the hospital's growth plans the following summer.

hospital, Paul Balcom took the opportunity to praise the "tremendous talent and commitment" of his staff. His views were seconded by LCH's Chaplain Fr. Frank Lawler, O F M, who said he found the hospital was "not just a faceless institution but rather a lot of concerned people," who cared for their patients as individuals.

This concern for the individual was reflected in specialized centers, which addressed special needs. One of the fastest-growing areas of the hospital was the rehabilitation center. A medical field that developed in the years following World War II to meet the needs of injured veterans, rehabilitation also served the needs of hundreds of victims disabled by infantile paralysis, stroke, and major injuries. Concern for those with limited physical abilities enlarged the scope of rehabilitation.

The traditional response to loss of function through stroke, spinal cord injury, or other causes has usually been to compensate and work around it, but the staff at the center often used a more positive approach. Patients were carefully assessed by a multidisciplinary team directed by Dr. Robert Marks, a physiatrist specializing in physical medicine and rehabilitation and the program's first Medical Director. Starting in many cases with total immobility, patients can develop life skills to increase independence. Sitting up, balancing, and weight-bearing are steps toward mobility. The confidence inspired by caring personnel has allowed paraplegics mobility through operating motorized wheelchairs. Others who were once wheelchair-bound have progressed to being pedestrians.

With determination, some reach goals like bowling, hiking, and golf.

Specialists work together to develop strength and cope with changes. Inpatient treatment is often followed by outpatient reinforcement, which continues therapy with greater convenience.

Touching stories of recovery unfold daily at the center. The patients and the rehabilitation team have faith in one other; their confidence in people's ability to meet challenges breeds hope and makes miracles occur often in the face of apparently insurmountable odds.

The idea that public education can improve public health is, in some ways, revolutionary. An aura of mystery has always surrounded the healing arts; recent advances in medical science have made the practice of medicine even more puzzling. Empowering ordinary people to keep themselves well requires confidence in the democratic system, and modern doctors have been willing to accept that challenge.

Lorain Community Hospital, in association with *The Lorain Journal*, sponsored public forums on health issues. The first seminar, in May, 1976, was held in the auditorium of Lorain High School before an overflow audience of over 1,000. Many of the audience were seated on the stage, as all the regular seats were filled! The first seminar was on stroke and elicited inquiries nationwide and front-page comment in *The Wall Street Journal*. A second program in October, 1976 addressed heart disease and was even more popular. The local newspaper was understandably proud of its role in this project. "Still, the real groundwork came back in June of

NOT QUITE A DISASTER

Every large-scale disaster that challenges a hospital shares certain characteristics: fear, concern, pain, and the reaction of a trained team of professionals rising to the challenge of an emergency. In early May, 1977, 110 junior high students aboard three buses were returning from a class trip to Washington, D. C. Suddenly, almost all of them developed frightening symptoms. Lorain Community and St. Joseph hospitals moved into high gear, summoning extra staff

1975 when Irving Leibowitz, editor of *The Lorain Journal*, was working on one of his Editor's Notebooks," a feature in the paper related. "The medical seminars were born with that column, which appeared June 29, 1975.

"'Here in Lorain County, the doctors of the medical society could perform a real public service by holding a series of seminars on illnesses and how to prevent them . . . There are thousands of people walking around with high blood pressure—the silent killer—who do not know it,' Leibowitz wrote.

"Later Leibowitz got together with Paul Balcom, executive director of Lorain Community Hospital, and the dream became reality. Together, they launched the first seminar on stroke last May [1976]. St. Joseph Hospital and Amherst Hospital added their resources for the October 13 seminar, both describing the seminars as valuable tools with which to enlarge the scope of their aims—the good health of the public."

Over 1,200 people crowded the Admiral King High School auditorium on a fall day to listen to their local cardiologists discuss heart disease. Dr. Denis Radefeld moderated a panel of three heart specialists, Dr. Razak Kherani, Dr. Thomas Sfiligoj, and Dr. John Schaeffer. Their presentations and answers to questions presented by the audience were professional and informative.

The following year, LCH received an award from the Ohio Hospital Association for presenting the initial seminar on stroke. The

Better and Better:
Leadership in the Growing Years

and utilizing emergency-
trained teams to screen and
treat the sick and
frightened youngsters. At
their home in Port Clinton,
the students' waiting
parents were told of the
mini-epidemic. Once the
symptoms were treated,
they seemed to vanish as
quickly as they came.
Only one student was
actually hospitalized at
LCH, but the memory of
the dramatic hospital visit
at the end of their school
trip probably remained
with every student for
years to come.

following May, a seminar on cancer was scheduled; a worthwhile tradition had begun.

The piece of equipment that had so impressed James Bardoner when he first joined the Board was finally installed in July, 1976. It was called a delta scanner, but the acronym for its function—computerized axial tomography—caused most people to refer to it as a CAT scanner. This new technology was hailed worldwide as the most significant development since the discovery of x-rays at the turn of the century. Combining the diagnostic abilities of an x-ray enhanced with the analytic speed of a computer, the process allowed imaging that could detect differences in tissue mass, showing abnormalities in areas previously hidden except to exploratory surgery.

More than a single machine, the scanner was a complex system of computers, cameras, shields, and other equipment that was housed in three rooms. Its intricacy required special training to operate and even more training to translate the myriad results recorded on monitors and reams of computer printout.

"The device is so advanced," a newspaper story reported, "that the hospital has established an educational committee comprised of physicians, surgeons, radiologists and hospital administrators to implement an 'intensified orientation, so we don't have misuse or abuse,' according to the hospital's executive director, Paul Balcom."

While the equipment required extra training for the technicians, it made the testing much simpler for the patients. To them, the procedure was similar to having a photo taken: a time-consuming, elaborate photograph. Since the scanner distinguished between densities—fat, fluid, tissue, and tumor—many complicated, painful, and duplicating procedures could be eliminated. In six months, the system was used on over 600 patients, making many earlier routine tests and invasive procedures unnecessary while both enhancing the quality of medicine and reducing medical costs. The reduced cost of diagnosis made the substantial price tag on the scanner cost-effective. The total outlay of $575,000 was partially covered by a $25,000 grant from the James R. Nicholl Foundation of Amherst. Lorain Community Hospital was proud of its impressive new machinery and felt the large expenditure was justified. There was, however, a general feeling that many hospitals considered themselves in a competition to acquire as many "new toys" as possible and that this tendency drove up costs.

The Lorain Journal assured its readers that this was not the case, in an editorial titled "Hospital Scanner Needed." The editor applauded lack of duplication; the nearest scanners were located in Cleveland and Akron, and there was complete cooperation among local hospitals in using the one at LCH. Scheduling and even transportation of patients were being arranged for the most economical use of the modern miracle. It was the best answer, the paper concluded, prophesying that "the time will come when a scanner will be standard equipment in every hospital."

Better and Better:
Leadership in the Growing Years

The Lakeland Institute, the Alcoholism and Chemical Dependency Treatment Center of LCH, had grown as information and understanding about the nature of alcoholism and chemical dependencies expanded. In response to the needs of society, the hospital examined its facilities and modified them to suit the needs of the patients served. It was observed that all patients did not fit the same profile; they differed widely in age and education, for example. This resulted in a commitment to further study as well as to individualize treatment. The special facility had the benefit of constant checking by the Board on care and results. The program was cited

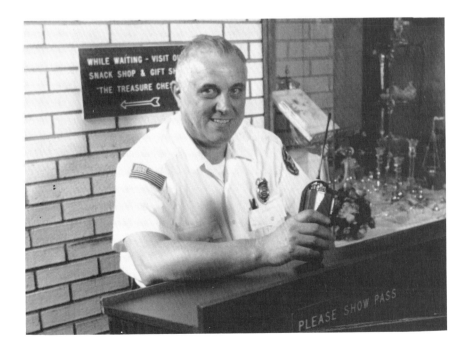

Security officer Horst Kuehne welcomes visitors to LCH.

as one of the top 100 treatment programs in the nation by independent assessors.

Early in 1979, the hospital Board announced plans for a $20 million expansion to increase the number of hospital beds to accommodate the growing Great Lakes Comprehensive Rehabilitation Center. The expansion would also include therapy areas and provide for a new emergency-ambulatory care department, construction of an attached private-practice medical office building, and construction of a free-standing alcohol and chemical dependency center to be designated The Lakeland Institute. A major feature of this plan was a designated nine-bed alcohol detoxification unit to be housed in the hospital proper, separate from the psychiatric department.

There was competition for the expanded alcohol treatment program from eight greater Cleveland hospitals since only one demonstration center was to be constructed in northeast Ohio. Additionally, there was protest from other hospitals over the plans for additional beds, general and rehabilitation. They claimed that since they were operating below full capacity, there was no need for LCH to expand. For almost a year, meetings and studies were held, with the strong possibility that the certificate of need required by the Ohio State Health Department would be denied for some or all of the major expansion plans. By year's end, however, a compromise was reached. The program was scaled down. The number of beds would not grow at LCH, but some existing beds would be devoted to specialized rehabilitation use. An editorial appearing in *The Lorain Journal* lauded the arrangement as "a better plan. By tailoring expansion dreams to the times, the Lorain Community Directors have proven themselves to be good administrators—and good citizens." Lakeland Institute was approved by the state as was a similar unit in Metropolitan General in Cleveland. The medical office building was also approved.

The hospital's 1979 annual report was able to boast of fifteen years of "quality care with fiscal responsibility," citing the two successful major expansion plans: planned future construction of a fifty-bed free-standing residential alcoholism-chemical-treatment center, modernization of the main hospital, and contracting to build a medical office building. When the hospital's site had been chosen more than fifteen years earlier, there was room for considerable expansion, and it became progressively obvious that the hospital's founders and original planners had envisioned the future very well. A well-designed office complex is useful in recruiting new physicians; inevitably, it increases hospital use.

The plans for Lakeland Medical Center had been unveiled in the spring of 1977. The design featured an open-air effect in an atrium surrounded by three floors of office suites. It was engineered to be built gradually; the first floor, with just over a dozen offices, would be ready initially, with the structure growing gradually to a total of 26 doctors' suites with adjacent space available for future growth.

*Aerial of Lorain
Community Hospital
in 1982, showing
construction of the
rehabilitation center
and cafeteria.*

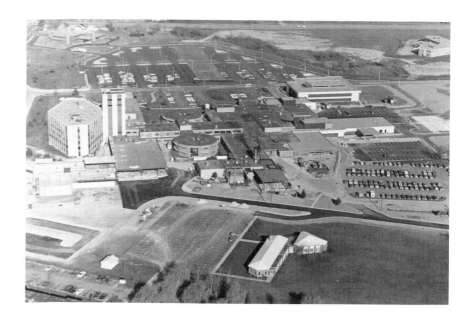

CHAPTER SIX

Challenge of Maturity: Improving and Specializing

The early eighties were not kind to Lorain. The recession that hit the whole country seemed to have struck hardest at the manufacturing centers of the Midwest. Work at local major plants was sporadic; unemployment, with its attendant social evils, became a key local concern, with area unemployment hitting a high of 25 percent.

Lorain Community Hospital entered this difficult decade as a good corporate citizen. On one hand, it remained one of the largest locally owned and managed businesses in the area. The hospital provided jobs, met payrolls, acted as a responsible tenant for the city's property, and served as a continuing feature in Lorain's menu of attractions for new business. It also made a concerted effort to meet the challenges born of a difficult economic period.

Two ways in which the hospital responded to less-than-ideal times were typical of the philosophy that had always guided it. The first was to pledge itself to continue its high standards. In January, 1980, the Joint Commission on Accreditation of Hospitals awarded a two-year accreditation to the hospital that declared it had "set forth optimal

achievable goals of excellence against which a facility can measure itself."
It was pointed out that meeting these criteria, which are considerably
higher than government standards, is voluntary.

The second approach was to create programs that were closely
attuned with the changing needs of the community. Projects ranged from
"Operation Preview," which prepared children for hospital stays by
making them familiar with the equipment, staff, and daily routine in a
hospital, to an exercise circuit, Parcourse, on the hospital grounds to

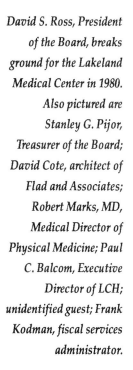

David S. Ross, President of the Board, breaks ground for the Lakeland Medical Center in 1980. Also pictured are Stanley G. Pijor, Treasurer of the Board; David Cote, architect of Flad and Associates; Robert Marks, MD, Medical Director of Physical Medicine; Paul C. Balcom, Executive Director of LCH; unidentified guest; Frank Kodman, fiscal services administrator.

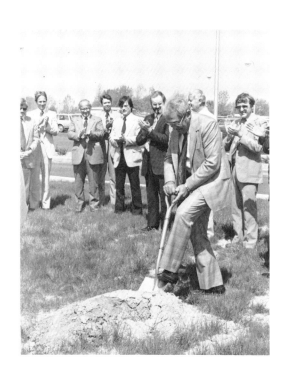

Challenge of Maturity:
Improving and Specializing

encourage healthful lifestyles in stressful times. Another continuing program, expanded from its inception in 1974, was "Make Today Count," a support group for families and individuals experiencing life-threatening illness. They shared common concerns and gained strength to deal with

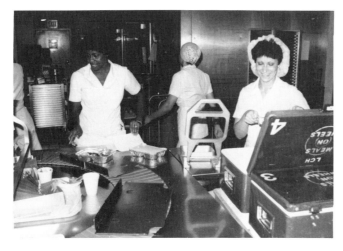

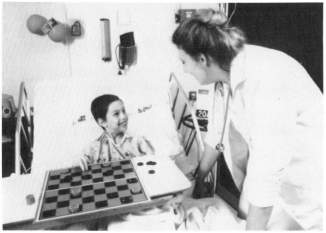

Lillian Green and Gladys Torres pack meals for the Meals on Wheels program, 1986.

Patient well-being has always been a priority for LCH, especially for children. Beginning with "operation preview" on February 9, 1980, children who were soon to be admitted to the hospital could be given a preview of the hospital.

*Anna Hickey operates
LCH's first digital
subtraction angiography
in 1982.*

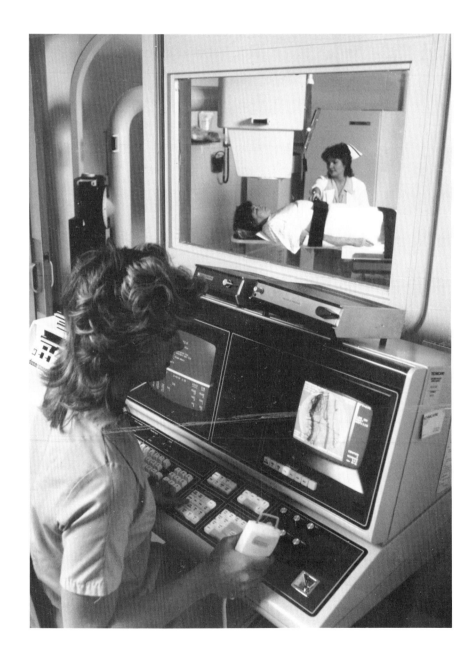

Challenge of Maturity:
Improving and Specializing

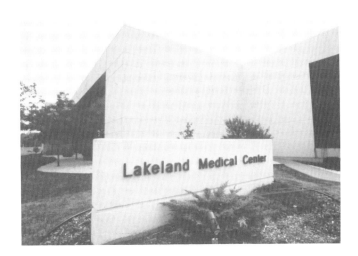

Lakeland Medical Center combines physician offices and classrooms for LCH's educational programs.

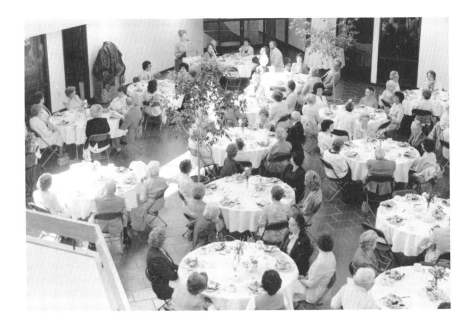

A LCH auxiliary luncheon held in the Lakeland Medical Center, May, 1982. The beautiful surroundings offered in the atrium of the building have welcomed seminars, fashion shows, even a beautiful wedding, and many other events through the years.

their own situations.

Many older Americans dimly remember when doctors made house calls. Over the years, this method of health care delivery was gradually deemed impractical. The doctor spent valuable time in transit; important equipment and diagnostic tools were only available in the office or hospital. In time, the home visit became a rosy memory, with the reality of less-than-optimum health service obscured. But as the cycle of medical administration turned, the high cost of facilities caused hospital leaders to reexamine their policies. Health care had long ceased to be the exclusive province of the family doctor; a wide range of specialists now offered treatment, therapy, and other individualized services. Perhaps, it was

The opening of the new emergency care center, December, 1981 (left to right, back to front): Mayor Joseph Zahorec, Paul Balcom, Denis Radefeld, MD, Governor James Rhodes, and David Ross.

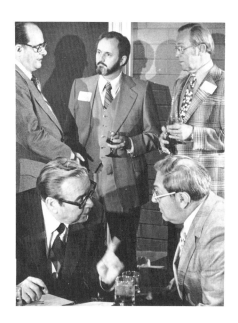

argued, there were times when centralized health care was not the best route, either economically, or more important, in terms of the patient.

As Paul Balcom wrote in 1983, it sometimes became wise "to defer or eliminate the need for more expensive inpatient hospital care in situations when the patient can otherwise receive the same treatment away from the hospital setting." Historically, it was a return, with important modifications, to house calls. At that time, Lorain Community Hospital became the first hospital in Lorain County to offer a Medicare-approved, hospital-based home health care service.

In the rehabilitation sphere, for example, physically challenged patients who would be exhausted just getting to a hospital for treatment

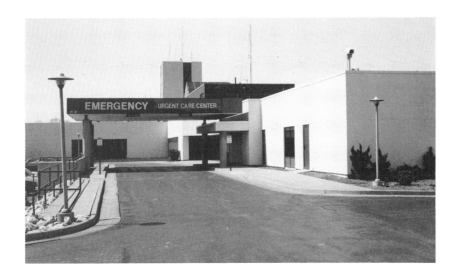

The Urgent Care Center began receiving patients in 1983. In 1989, LCH invested $1.7 million to upgrade its emergency facilities to qualify for Level II trauma care. Level II trauma facilities must have a team of specially trained nurses and an emergency-room physician on twenty-four-hour duty. Trauma surgeons, anesthesiologists, and operating-room nurses must be available within thirty minutes.

were visited by specialists. "We teach people to get around in their homes," explained physical therapist Joyce Hill in a *Lorain Journal* article on home health services. Working out patients' problems in their own environments, she pointed out, seemed more practical and realistic than the most elaborate treatment center. Returning to self-sufficiency meant a patient would not need to be sent to an expensive nursing home. But there were more important concerns than cost; providing independence to a challenged person afforded a quality of life that could not be measured in dollars.

Since its inauguration in 1976, the rehabilitation program had grown steadily at Lorain Community Hospital. It was a proud day when

Since its opening in 1976, Lorain Community Hospital's Great Lakes Regional Rehabilitation Center has gained wide recognition for its quality services from northern Ohio hospitals, health agencies, and health-care professionals. It received full accreditation for its program of physical rehabilitation from the nationally recognized accreditation body for rehab facilities, the Commission on Accreditation of Rehabilitation Facilities.

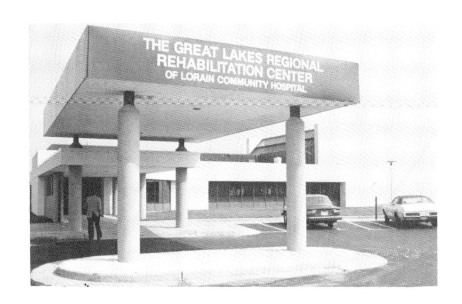

the hospital hosted Nobel prize nominee Dr. Howard Rusk at an open house on October 16, 1982. As the "father of rehabilitation medicine," Dr. Rusk could join in the pride of the 300 guests as they admired the new Great Lakes Regional Rehabilitation Center facility. His speech was a graceful tribute to the staff and supporters of the center, describing the progress in the field and its contributions to improving the human condition. He told the story of Louis Pasteur, father of immunization, who suffered a stroke in his forties and went on to make his greatest discoveries in the last twenty-five years of life. Quoting the famous scientist, he said, "The future belongs to those who accomplish most for suffering humanity." Copies of Dr. Rusk's autobiography, *A World To Care For*, were

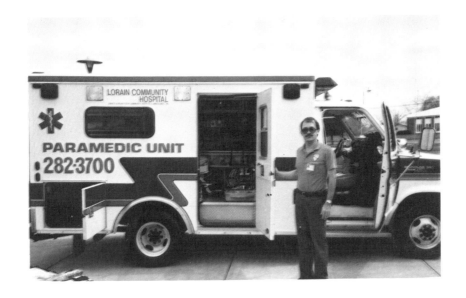

Brent Russell proudly presents LCH's paramedic unit.

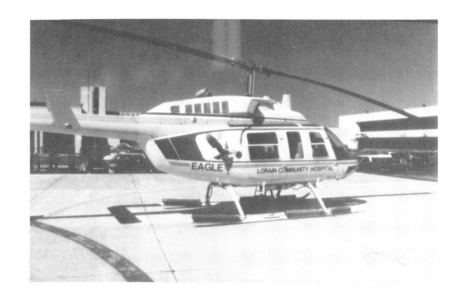

While it was invaluable in saving lives, the EAGLE, LCH's rescue-helicopter service, was discontinued after two years of service on December 31,1985. With an annual expense of $750,000, the cost for operating the service was just too high.

Nurse manager Julia Meeks pauses at the nurses' station during one of its quieter moments.

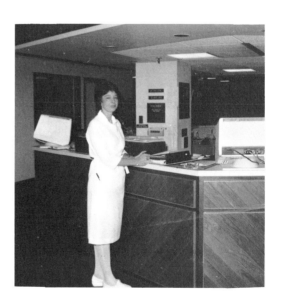

given to all in attendance. The Center, one of only eight comprehensive hospital-based rehabilitation centers in Ohio, enjoys a regional reputation.

In 1981, the long-awaited Lakeland Medical Center opened its doors. Designed by Flad and Associates of Madison, Wisconsin, it was immediately hailed as an architectural landmark, receiving an award for excellence from the American Institute of Architects. The general contractor was a local firm, Elmer Hume of Amherst. The multilevel building featured an open, glassed atrium, lavishly planted with full-sized trees. This cheerful area served as an additional waiting room for the private-practice offices that overlooked it. The atrium was also designed as the site of mini-health seminars, fashion shows, and social events.

The Lakeland Institute's new building was also honored for its design. In addition, its alcoholism treatment program was designated by the state of Ohio as a model treatment facility for the state. The program consisted of detoxification and psychosocial assessment in the hospital, followed by twenty-eight days of residential treatment at the fifty-bed center. The residential program was followed up with a one-year outpatient treatment period.

In 1984, after years of preparation and planning, the hospital felt it had all the ingredients to initiate a full trauma program. Years of successful operation of rescue units, hundreds of patients cared for under trying conditions in emergency rooms, and thousands of dollars expended on special equipment added up to the reality of presenting to the

THE COUNTY'S FIRST CAT SCANNER

When LCH acquired the county's first CAT scanner in 1976, *The Lorain Journal* prophesied that someday the sophisticated device would be standard in every hospital. In an article a short half-dozen years later, Paul Balcom described that future as the present. Both Elyria Memorial and St. Joseph hospitals planned their own units, based on the incredible success of the LCH system, which they had shared for four years. LCH endorsed these acquisitions to the Regional Planning Agency. Cooperation allowed them to acquire equipment previously thought available only to big-city hospitals.

community a modern trauma center.

Trauma, the medical term for injury, usually implies a serious multisystem problem requiring immediate and critical medical intervention followed by comprehensive clinical-resource availability on premises. Accidents of various kinds are a leading cause of death in the United States; they cause an even greater number of permanent disabilities. Before the science of trauma management was developed, many people died unnecessarily because of a lack of know-how and ability in handling patients in difficult straits. A relatively new area, trauma management quickly evolved as life-support skills and state-of-the-art equipment were combined with the will to meet the challenge.

Lorain Community Hospital, with its twenty-year tradition of serving the community, put together a team of surgeons, anesthesiologists, physicians, nurses, and clinical assistants to provide aggressive life-saving treatment around the clock. Surgical suites had been renovated and modernized. The newly upgraded rehabilitation center was available, with its own specially trained people. Consultants from the Emergency Medical Services Association and the Maryland Institute for Emergency Medical Services Systems provided expertise and guidelines.

LCH had been providing group-based paramedic rescue services following closure of the Lorain City Rescue Service, despite a $70,000 grant to the City of Lorain from the Lorain Community Hospital Auxiliary. However, most dramatic was the introduction of EAGLE, a fully equipped

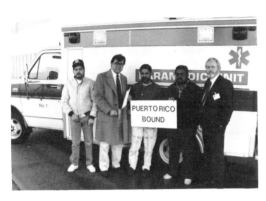

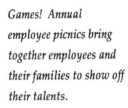

After a hurricane devastated Puerto Rico, Lorain Community Hospital assisted a community in need by donating a fully-equiped paramedic unit ambulance.

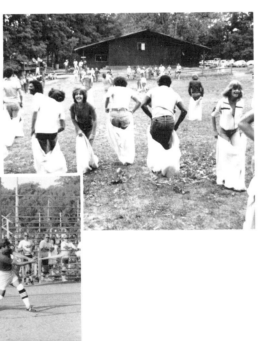

Games! Annual employee picnics bring together employees and their families to show off their talents.

Staffers recalled sometimes seeing deer wandering in the nearby golf course in winter, but they never expected one to venture close to the hospital. Three days before Christmas, 1984, however, a confused doe crashed into the hospital's medical records office. The 200-pound deer alarmed weekend workers and created havoc when it jumped through the plate glass window.

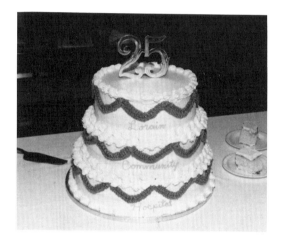

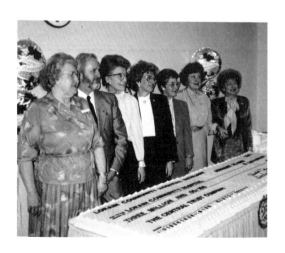

Challenge of Maturity:
Improving and Specializing

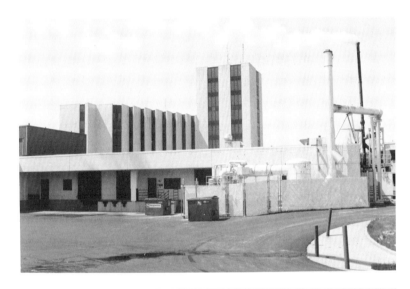

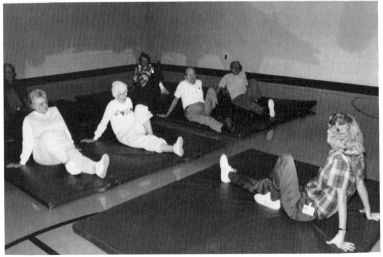

advance life-support helicopter service staffed by a paramedic (EMT-A) and a trauma nurse functioning under the direction of a certified physician director. The aircraft was equipped with a communications network to link field paramedics with emergency room physicians. EAGLE (an acronym for Emergency Assistance to Ground and Lake Environments) quickly caught the imagination of the north central Ohio area. The EAGLE visited many schools and other sites to demonstrate its value to the area. The EAGLE staff worked closely with the area rescue squads providing education, support, and communication. While most of the flights concerned unfortunate victims of misadventure, on one occasion the EAGLE served as a stork, providing emergency care to an expectant mother in Sheffield Village. When Geri Darmos discovered her baby was arriving ahead of schedule, her husband called the rescue squad; they in turn summoned the helicopter. The original plan to fly the mother to a Cleveland hospital was again thwarted by the impatient youngster. The delivery was performed by flight nurse Cindy Lowther in the city park, where the craft had landed to pick up the patient. "It's kind of nice to go to a scene where it's good news instead of sad," was the nurse's observation.

For almost two years the EAGLE program was commended for its life-saving activities. Tales of gallant rescue were related. Mayor Hobart Johnson of Vermilion praised contingency plans for air evacuation arranged when parts of his town were isolated by bridge closures while under repair. When a Toledo emergency helicopter crashed, LCH immediately offered the use of its equipment to St. Vincent's Hospital as that city coped with its tragedy. But while the benefits were impressive, the expenses were staggering. In the face of cost-cutting measures by Medicare, Medicaid, and other insurance carriers, Paul Balcom realized that services would have to be reduced throughout the hospital. The dramatic single rescues would have to be sacrificed to the mundane expenditures that saved and mended scores of lives every day. The EAGLE folded its rotors at the end of 1985.

That same year saw continued concern over the possibilities of ecological damage to the hospital because of the city's intent to reroute a sewer line near the hospital. The issue had caused some friction between the hospital and Lorain's City Council in 1984, but the two organizations

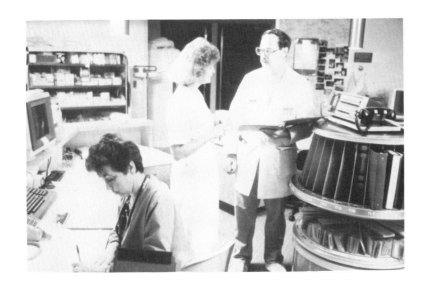

James Andrasko, M. D., confers with Sophie Beckler, R. N., in the critical care center. Seated is Barbara Permelia, R. N.

were, nonetheless, united in their concern for the good of the community.

The hospital was able to refinance its revenue bonds from 1968, 1969, and 1981 with the approval of the City Council in the fall of 1985. "Tax-free bonds may be re-financed twice. We lowered our interest rate from 12 percent to 9.75 percent, saving a lot of money," said Paul Balcom. "McDonald & Company Securities underwrote the issue. The bonds were rated A- by Standard & Poor's."

"Both council [and Lorain mayor William Parker] realize the hospital could save $137,000 a year in interest payments in each of the next

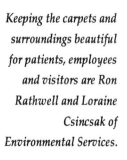

Keeping the carpets and surroundings beautiful for patients, employees and visitors are Ron Rathwell and Loraine Csincsak of Environmental Services.

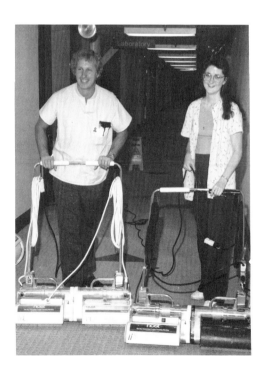

THE LAKELAND HEALTH CARE CORPORATION ORGANIZATIONAL CHART

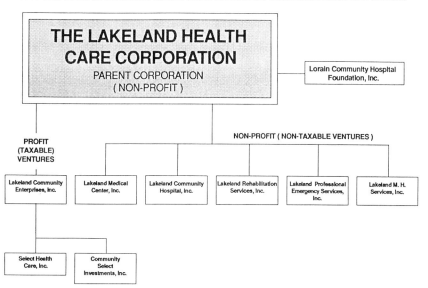

27 years through refinancing its bonds at today's lower interest rates," *The Lorain Journal* pointed out in a 1985 editorial.

Lorain Community Hospital entered its third decade as a diversified health care leader. In 1984, James L. Bardoner became the new Chairman of the Board of Trustees, and the organization was corporately restructured. Corporate titles were modified to accommodate the new structure. A holding company was established, along with an impressive litany of affiliate companies, created to contribute a wide range of services for the community. They included: The Lakeland Health Care Corporation (the parent), Lakeland Community Hospital, Inc., Lorain Community Hospital Foundation, Inc., Community Hospitals Ambulance,

DR. COSTIN:

"THE TRUE MIRACLE OF

SURGERY IS THE

BODY'S HEALING

PROCESS. ALL THE

SURGEON CAN TRY TO

DO IS MAKE REPAIRS

WITHOUT DISRUPTING

THE TISSUES TOO

MUCH."

Inc., Lakeland Community Enterprises, Inc., Select Health Care Equipment, Inc., Lakeland Medical Center, Inc., Lakeland Professional Services, Inc., Select Health Care, Inc., Select Communications, Inc., and Community Select Investments, Inc. The impressive list of companies only hinted at the actual people-oriented services they supported. For example, Select Health Care Equipment, Inc., helped patients and their families locate and select equipment, supplies, and professional services from an ever-increasing array of health care products to be used in the home. The days of borrowing Aunt Millie's old hospital bed or wheelchair "for the duration" had vanished in an avalanche of specialized equipment and supplies, which, while their variety guaranteed superior service, sometimes left the layman confused.

Cardiologist John Schaeffer, M. D., is assisted by Leslie Zeck, R. N., in the cardiac catheterization laboratory. Angie Knittle operates the equipment from inside the booth.

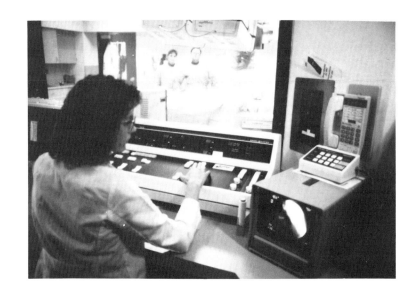

Since its opening days, Lorain Community Hospital had offered a broad range of services to people afflicted with diabetes. This disease, long unrecognized by much of the population, was first diagnosed in 3000 B. C. Over the centuries, treatment was flawed due to ignorance of the underlying cause: the failure of the pancreas to produce insulin, which

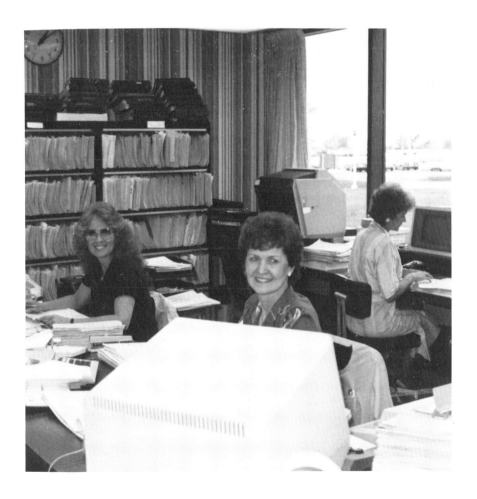

Accurate record-keeping is important for the successful operation of the hospital: Sharon Miller, Darlene Klingenmeier, Paulette Wolfe, of the patient accounting department, 1988.

stores and burns sugar in the blood. The discovery, isolation, and eventual use of insulin in treating diabetes began in the 1920s. Remarkable advances were made in the years following: precise testing methods, a variety of insulin types, and treatments to prevent vision loss in diabetic patients. Successful treatment for this disease demands a high level of education, monitoring, and support. The hospital had created many programs to meet these needs, and in June, 1986, the Diabetes Comprehensive Care Center was opened. Dr. Patricio Aycinena, an endocrinologist who was soon to be certified by the American Diabetes Association, was recruited by LCH to direct a team of registered nurses,

Designed by LCH's Health Resource Center, the Parcourse is a 1.25-mile self-guided fitness circuit. The Parcourse opened in March, 1987 and is available to area residents free of charge.

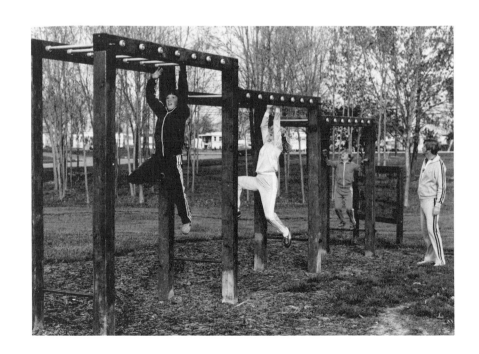

Challenge of Maturity:
Improving and Specializing

dietitians, pharmacists, physical therapists, and social workers. The emphasis of the program was continuing education, diet, exercise, and medical programs, under the individual care of the patient's own doctor. Since Medicare policies often dictated shorter hospital stays, many patients were without the information they needed to maintain good health and prevent diabetic-related medical complications. The specialized center was created, as Paul Balcom explained, to "fill a void for the newly diagnosed diabetic, diabetics being changed to insulin use and/or diabetics needing education."

In October, 1988, a *Chronicle-Telegram* feature announced that Lorain Community Hospital, St. Joseph Hospital, and Elyria Memorial Hospital planned to work closely to share more facilities and avoid duplication. As Paul Balcom explained, "We're going to mutually support each other and see how we can enhance one another." The plan included sharing equipment through patient referrals from a "home base" hospital to another facility for a special treatment or test if necessary. While the hospitals had always publicly displayed a certain degree of competitiveness, cooperation had existed for years at many levels: LCH had offered use of its CAT scanner to neighbor institutions since its installation; Elyria Memorial Hospital made use of St. Joseph's laundry facilities; and LCH and St. Joseph used Elyria's cardiac catheterization services. Though the three hospitals considered themselves successful even in a difficult economic period, they realized the predictable economic constraints in the world would provide strong incentives to adopt efficient procedures that were consistent with quality care, including cooperating and collaborating with one other, including even the ultimate possibility of institutional consolidation.

As President and CEO, Paul Balcom had promised early in the economic downturn, the hospital had responded to the needs of the community. It had grown to meet new challenges; it had acknowledged that, in good times or bad, individuals and cities needed and deserved help in times of distress. He promised that while the hospital would adjust itself to the times, its goal would not change:

"We will implement innovative developments. Opportunities for more self-help and an awareness of the need to foster wellness concepts will be identified, as opposed to primarily focusing on the issues of illness, as we have done in the past. Increasing emphasis will be given to the use of alternative forms of care. More testing will be required of patients prior to entering the hospital; stays will be shortened; outpatient services, home health services, or more care in the physician's office will become the trend.

"We need to use our health and human resources wisely during these generally difficult times, while simultaneously exercising all possible effort to revitalizing our general economy."

Those words, spoken in 1982, became even more relevant as a new decade unfolded. The nineties saw a drop in Lorain's population and continued uncertainty in its economic life, but the community and its community hospital were still committed to excellence.

THE FINANCIAL GROWTH OF LORAIN COMMUNITY HOSPITAL

LORAIN COMMUNITY HOSPITAL
EARLY BALANCE SHEET

December 1968

ASSETS

December 1968

LIABILITIES AND FUND BALANCE

Cash and Cash Equivalents	210,669	Accounts Payable	209,755
Investments and Limited Assets	122,822	Accrued Payroll and Taxes Withheld	98,694
Patient Accounts Receivable (Net)	388,634	Deferred Reimbursement 3rd Party	113,600
Receivable from 3rd Party Payors	129,170	Other Liabilities	10,613
Other Receivables (Net)	943		
Inventories	74,472		
Other Assets	18,993	Long Term Debt	2,982,594
Net Property, Plant & Equipment	3,360,905	Total Liabilities	3,415,256
		Fund Balance	891,352
Total General Fund Assets	4,306,608	Total Fund Balance & Liabilities	4,306,608

LORAIN COMMUNITY HOSPITAL
BALANCE SHEET
DECEMBER 31, 1992

December 1992

ASSETS

Cash and Cash Equivalents	4,847,486	Accounts Payable	2,609,079
Investments and Limited Assets	14,585,785	Accrued Payroll/Taxes Withheld	2,103,129
Patient Accounts Receivable (Net)	9,553,034	Deferred Reimbursement 3rd Party	310,877
Receivable from 3rd Party Payors	1,455,119	Other Liabilities	1,078,207
Other Receivables (Net)	372,217		
Inventories	441,197		
Other Assets	1,969,861	Long Term Debt	28,109,680
Net Property, Plant & Equipment	29,641,405	Total Liabilities	34,210,972
		Fund Balance	28,655,132
Total General Fund Assets	62,866,104	Total Fund Balance & Liabilities	62,866,104

December 1992

LIABILITIES AND FUND BALANCE

AFFILIATIONS AND ACCREDITATIONS

AFFILIATIONS:
University Hospitals of Cleveland

ACCREDITATIONS:
Joint Commission on Accreditation of Healthcare Organizations (JCAHO)
Commission on Accreditation of Rehabilitation of
        Rehabilitation Facilities (CARF)
College of American Pathologists (CAP) Laboratory Accreditation
American Association of Blood Banks
Nuclear Regulatory Commission
American College of Radiologists
        Accreditation of Radiologists
        Accreditation of Mammography Suite
Ohio Department of Health
Ohio Department of Mental Health
American College of Surgeons Commission on Cancer
American Diabetic Association
Medicare and Medicaid

TEACHING AFFILIATIONS:
Ashland University
Baldwin-Wallace College
Bowling Green/Medical College of Ohio
Case Western Reserve University
Cincinnati University
Cleveland State University
Cuyahoga Community College
Delta College
Dominican College of New York
Fairview Family Practitioner Program
John Carroll University
Lorain County Community College
Lorain County Joint Vocational School
Methodist Theological School in Ohio
Oberlin College
Ohio State University
Providence Hospital
Sandusky Providence
University of Akron
University of Toledo

*Since 1973, the
Lakeland Institute
has been one of the
most recognized
chemical dependency
programs in Ohio
and the region. The
institute was
designated by the
state of Ohio as a
model treatment
facility.*

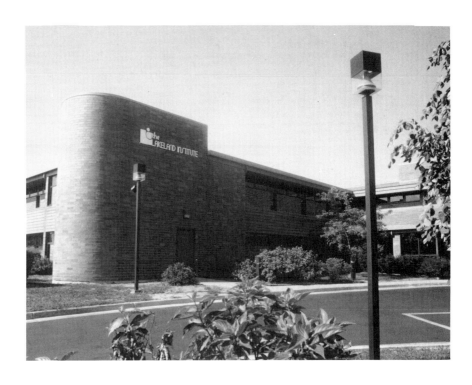

CHAPTER SEVEN

The Journey Continues: Approaching the Millennium

To read the daily newspaper is to be aware of the challenges a hospital faces in the last decade of the twentieth century. There are the mysterious—sometimes frightening—developments of "new" diseases and the painstaking, cutting-edge research that identifies and begins to control them and to bring help to sick people and greater health to healthy people. There are the heart-wrenching tales of illness and trauma that afflict mankind, from the individual tragic accident to the tidal waves of misery generated by wars and natural disasters.

There are triumphs as well—an almost scriptural quality to stories where "the blind see, the lame walk"; terms like "neuro-ophthalmology" and "hip-replacement surgery" only add a modern luster to what many accept as miraculous.

In every section of the newspaper are stories about health care: the business section describes the soaring cost of hospital equipment and the efforts of hospitals to pare costs while maintaining quality. The human-interest section features the graying of America: 80 percent of the country's health care costs relate to services rendered to citizens in the final two years

Fourteen "Windows to the Future," made of hand-crafted, beveled, leaded glass, were installed by designer and craftsman Mark Cavanaugh, Jr., and Mark Cavanaugh, Sr., of Cavanaugh Glass. The glass was installed in the lobby in December, 1990 in recognition of major benefactors to LCH following a $2 million fundraising effort by the Hospital Foundation.

John A. Costin, M. D. Neuro-Ophthalmologist, started the Regional Eye Program at Lorain Community Hospital in 1979. Using technology such as the Argon-Krypton and YAG lasers, most eye surgery can now be done on an outpatient basis.

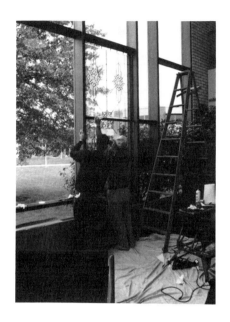

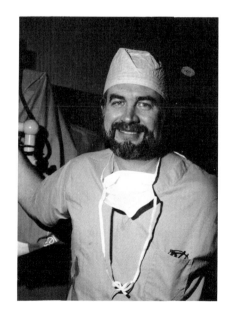

The Journey Continues:
Approaching the Millennium

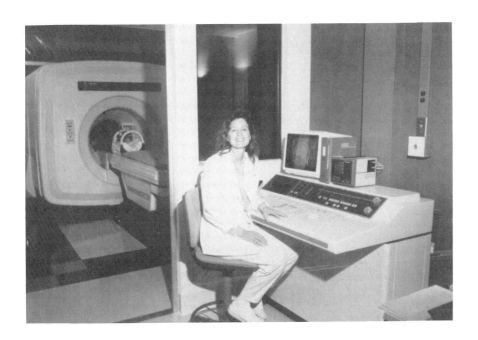

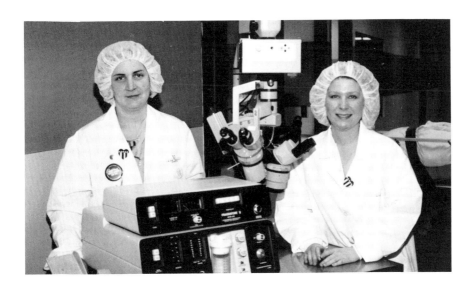

A magnetic resonance imaging system was installed at LCH in May 1992 as a first hospital-based unit in Lorain County.

Optical equipment used to repair trauma to the eye was loaned to an allied hospital in Saudi Arabia during Operation Desert Storm on January 28, 1991. The request for the loan was made by Camille Rhodehamel, R. N., a first lieutenant reservist who served with the 350th EVAC unit in Saudi Arabia. Prior to her service in Saudi Arabia, Rhodehamel was a part of the LCH surgical department team. Two days following the request, the final plans for the equipment's shipment were made. "LCH has a history of willingness to help and a reputation for doing what is takes to get the job done," said Paul Balcom. "Camille knew she could count on us." Debbie Eldridge and Terri Gay prepare equipment for its transport.

of their lives, when those lives have been extended, in part, through medical advances. The front page banners the government's efforts to understand—and solve—the gigantic problems of America's health care system. The editorial page attacks the problem on a local level.

Lorain Community Hospital may not be named in each of these stories, yet its people—staff, patients, friends—are aware that their hospital makes news every day. Where disease and trauma threaten individual lives and families, the hospital steps in. From powerful MRI scans to

The opening of the cardiac catheterization laboratory in 1987 was a long-awaited event.

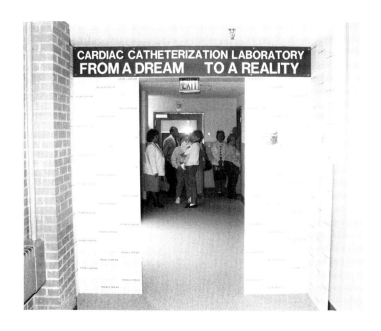

nonsurgical breast biopsy procedures, each patient is carefully diagnosed using appropriate state-of-the art technology that can reduce uncertainty and fear of the unknown. When major disasters threaten, LCH is ready, and not only local problems are addressed.

During the tense and dramatic days of January, 1992, the hospital lent special eye-surgery equipment to an allied hospital in Saudi Arabia as part of Operation Desert Storm. Anticipating possible ground-war injuries, the hospital estimated that 20 percent of the wounds would be eye-related.

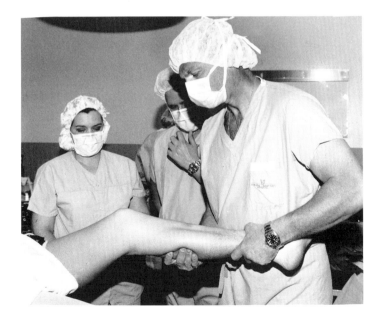

Dr. Michael Kolczun II , Orthopedic Surgeon examines a patient's knee prior to performing knee-joint replacement, 1993

This same concern for eye care led Dr. John Costin and his associates in Alcon Surgical, Inc., to devise procedures to enhance the safety and effectiveness of cataract surgery. LCH's Regional Eye Program, which started in 1979 under Dr. Costin, could boast its latest tool: the Argon-Krypton laser, which uses a narrow beam of light energy focused through a microscope to repair tears in the retina, seal off leaking blood vessels, and open holes in clouded membranes. This technology reduces what was once an extremely restrictive hospital stay to an outpatient

Located on the newly remodeled fourth floor of LCH, the Skilled Nursing Facility features private, comfortable rooms and care on a 24-hour basis.

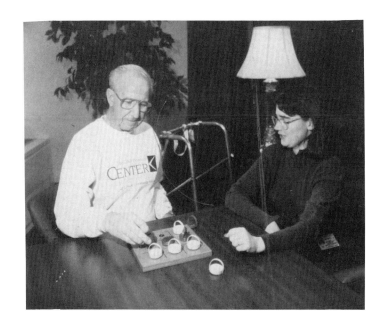

Pursuing the dream involves careful planning and teamwork. A 1988 finance committee included (left to right): Frank Kodman, Robert Capretto, Laurie Hoke, Stanley Pijor, Gerald Prucha, Ruth Calta, George Apolzon, Paul Driscol, and Paul Balcom.

President and Chief Executive Officer, Paul C. Balcom

surgery procedure. The savings in patient time, discomfort, and anxiety cannot be measured; the reduced cost of an extended hospital stay can easily be computed, as well as the reduced failure rate for this kind of operation. Comprehensive eye instrumentation constantly is added to the inventory.

In the late seventies, cardiac services at Lorain Community Hospital were limited; until the mid-seventies, there were no cardiologists, so internal medicine or family care physicians cared for cardiac patients. John Schaeffer, M. D., was the first formally trained and board certified cardiologist to affiliate (in 1976). Noninvasive cardiac testing, such as electrocardiograms, Holter monitoring, and stress tests became available, and the services grew. As new technologies presented themselves, a comprehensive cardiac rehabilitation program designed to help cardiac patients regain health and vitality was implemented in 1977. The open-heart surgery program at Elyria Memorial Hospital was endorsed by LCH as the singular operative unit to be developed in Lorain County.

Always striving to serve the patient better, LCH was bent on providing improved services in such an important area. People wanted to go to the hospital in their community for urgent cardiac services. January, 1987 saw the opening of a brand-new cardiac catheterization lab after a five-year struggle with the state that finally ended in LCH's favor. The new facility allowed all qualified cardiologists the opportunity to evaluate heart disease in their own community.

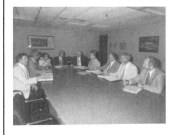
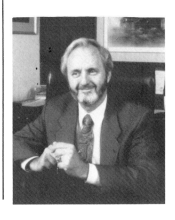

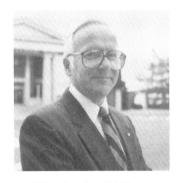

When Stanley G. Pijor was asked to be Treasurer of the hospital's Board of Trustees, he was a little shocked. "I figured a hospital of $3 million being built should have adequate working capital, right? I assumed that and accepted that position." The hospital started with working capital of only $35,000! He noted that during construction, in order to assure creditors, guarantees of $100,000 were needed from various business people in the community. "Most of those, like any other pledges—they were sure that they would not be called or needed. After the second year, we had no choice but to tell all the creditors or guarantors we have to have your money." However, most of the creditors were understanding. The hospital was able to get extended terms and got over its first hump. "That's how I got involved with it, and I have been overseeing the financial aspect of it for the last twenty-five years," Pijor said.

The improvements did not cease. Now there are ten cardiologists on permanent staff: Drs. Ismail Ahmed, Kenneth Bescak, Naim Farhat, Nelson Gencheff, David Grech, Senov Gursoy, Atol Hulyarkar, David Joyce, Patrick McGuinn, Stephen Moore, Charles O'Shaughnessy, Mohamad Salka, John Schaeffer, Michael Vacante, and Philip Wendschuch. The facility can do more than twenty various cardiac tests. Its latest addition is an intra-aorta balloon pump, a highly specialized piece of equipment that assists in heart function and increases the amount of blood the heart is able to pump. Dr. Schaeffer explained why these developments have been so important: "LCH has had tremendous foresight for the future treatment of coronary diseases. They are in tune with the needs of the medical community and responsive to the needs of the patients they serve."

Every hospital can attest to the multitudes of patients who enter their doors ailing from severe accident injuries, debilitating arthritis, spinal diseases, and fractures. LCH's orthopedic department has always been dedicated to helping people with these kinds of afflictions. Since LCH's Ohio Regional Center for Joint Implant Surgery opened in March, 1992, orthopedic surgeons have been performing in excess of 300 total joint replacements each year for patients throughout north central Ohio, and the program's medical director, Michael Kolczun II, M. D., is proud of the services it offers its patients.

"We offer the most up-to-date technology in a community hospital setting with more personalized care. We can do everything a larger facility

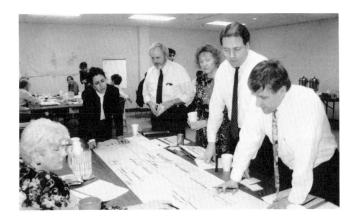

can do. Specifically, we do total hip, total knee, and total shoulder replacements."

The center, started by Dr. Kolczun and Dr. Donald Blanford, is "like a hospital within a hospital," with its own fourteen-bed unit and orthopedist-controlled staffing. The patient's comfort and well-being are paramount, and his or her recovery is monitored every step of the way under this comprehensive program. Dr. Blanford revealed why the center has done so well: "We enjoy a unique, good relationship at LCH among the medical staff, Board of Trustees, and Administration. The hospital was founded in response to the needs of the community and has continued that role. LCH is innovative in its technology and in its services. Service to the community has remained its primary goal." All qualified orthopedists on the LCH staff are invited to participate in the program.

January 25, 1993, bore witness to another opening at Lorain Community Hospital: that of the Skilled Nursing Facility. With sixteen

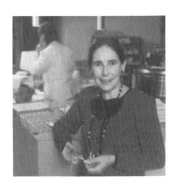

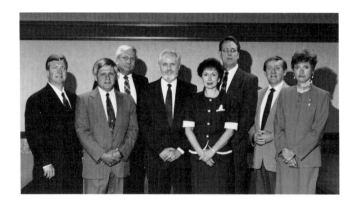

beds, the unit offers patients the quality care they need while in transitory phases of their recovery, whether they are waiting admittance into a rehabilitation center, need to build skills before they go home, or are waiting to be placed or returned to a nursing home. Knowing that external forces are often as important as internal forces in the process of healing, the caregivers at the Skilled Nursing Facility involve the patient's family and personal physician in the overall health program.

These directions show how Lorain Community Hospital, like most forward-looking health care institutions, is carefully evaluating all options to serve its patients and a growing list of corporate clients with both the high-quality care that they have come to expect, and the cost-conscious prudence that allows them to stay in business. It is hard for some to face the fact that though its mission may be humanitarian, a hospital's operation must be based on sound financial principles; it must compete in today's marketplace. The Board of Trustees of LCH, and especially its President, face these realities daily. In addition, the changing health-care climate requires constant surveillance; escalating costs and the American public's conviction that they deserve the best health care provide a constant dilemma, with considerable finger-pointing and confrontation when the system's delivery is less than perfect.

After James Bardoner's service of eight years as Chairman of the Hospital Board of Trustees, Vincent P. Traina became the new Chairman in 1992.

Traina explained the concerns of providing the latest services without aggravating rising costs. It is a dilemma with which the Board grapples continually. Keeping sight of what the health care industry is doing right helps curtail the bombardment of anxieties. He clarifies: "We are providing better and better health care. People are living to be older;

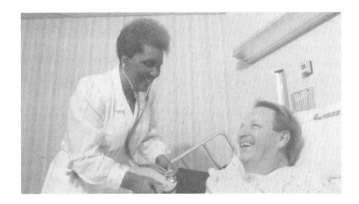

Vivian Charlton, R. N., takes time to share the good medicine of laughter with a patient.

not only that, but they are healthier later in life. This is a great tribute to our health care."

In the face of financial criticism of the system in general, LCH continues to serve the community as it has for the past twenty-nine years. Its record growth has allowed it to expand service offerings in a caring and cost-effective way. While every citizen is concerned about runaway inflation in the health care industry, those served by LCH can see that the hospital's expense-inflation rate has been less than half the national health care rate, with no loss of focus on quality of care, during the past five consecutive years.

"In many ways, health care is treated as an economic commodity," Paul Balcom points out. "It becomes subject to the laws of supply and demand. Demand, however, is measured in part on the basis of willingness

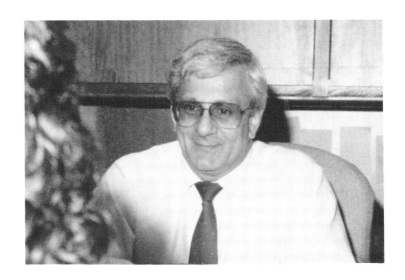

to purchase rather than on the patient's clinical need alone.

"The game plan is to provide appropriate, good-quality service at a competitive price. This approach means that some major changes will be made, but not to the point of qualitatively diminishing our end product."

Challenging times call for ingenuity and far-sightedness, and CEO Paul Balcom has won support from his peers and LCH staff for doing just that. Though the future may be unpredictable, many have faith in his guidance and leadership. Florencio Yuzon, M. D., among others, sang his praises: "Balcom is an excellent administrator. He has a very open mind on everything." Vincent Traina agrees, citing the emphasis placed on clear communications as the reason for LCH's positive outlook. His admiration for Balcom is evident: "He puts the cards on the table."

In facing the challenges of the future, Lorain Community Hospital is

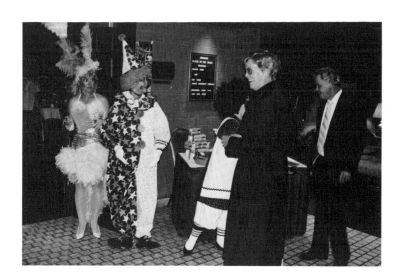

Supportive mental-health services are provided to employees through the employee assistance program. To provide outstanding healthcare service to the public, it is important that all the people involved in caring for patients feel good about themselves. Robert A. Capretto, Senior Vice President, lends an ear to an employee.

Costumed employees greet guests at the 1991 Service Awards Dinner.

113

A Service of Dedication
THE CRITICAL CARE CENTER
LORAIN COMMUNITY HOSPITAL
WEDNESDAY, MARCH 31, 1993

Almighty God, unto whom all hearts are open, all desires known, and from whom no secrets are hidden: Cleanse the thoughts of our hearts by the inspiration of Your Holy Spirit, that our dedication of this Critical Care Center may worthily magnify Your Name, we pray in the spirit of one known as the Great Physician—and the Good Shepherd.

The grace and peace of God be with all of you.

And also with you.

Almighty God, source of holiness and true purpose, it is right that we praise and glorify Your Name. Today we come before You to dedicate to Your service the Critical Care Center. Lord, may our prayer ascend from here as incense in Your sight so that Your blessings and graces come upon all who shall be admitted to this Unit.

Lord of Life, we are grateful for the wholesomeness of life and for the gift of good health.

Aware of the unity of body and spirit, we affirm our constant need for their harmony if we are to enjoy true health.

We are grateful for the marvels of medicine, for doctors and nurses, technicians and all who possess a healing touch and practice the art of healing.

We are thankful for the way in which our own bodies work to constantly heal themselves, restoring us to a state of health.

We acknowledge that we have been healed of depression and gloom by laughter and affection, healed of inner injury by the medicine of forgiveness; and for these times we are grateful as well.

As we rejoice in Your gift of health, may we be ever mindful of those who are steeped in sickness as part of the divine mystery of salvation.

We thank You for the presence in our lives of Your Son. In the ancient tradition of the prophets, He heralded and healed—both body and spirit—
in Your Sacred Name.

Blessed are You, Lord our God, who heals us and restores us to life.

As water is the symbol of refreshment and newness of life, so we bless each room; that all who come will be restored to wholeness and healing. If it should be time for the soul to leave the body, may we ever offer compassion and reverence. We ask this in Your Name.

Amen.

Delivered by Sister Noël Frey, R.S.M.
Director of Pastoral Services

well positioned for the recommended "managed-care" approach to health care reform. Described as a partnership between patient and primary-care physician, managed care is no stranger to LCH; since 1985, the hospital and many of its staff physicians have successfully operated a Physician Hospital Organization (PHO). This expertise will facilitate a smooth transition into this new philosophy of health care delivery, or managed health care as it is sometimes called. Total Quality Improvement is a program demonstrating the commitment of the hospital and its employees, Board, medical staff, and Auxiliary to the best service on a cost-effective basis; TQI is embraced by Lorain Community Hospital.

Musing on the changing health care picture, Balcom points out that some bargain-seeking purchasers will not choose LCH but others will, attracted by a demonstrated committment to provide quality health care at a fair and competitive price. He further notes that the hospital does not function in a vacuum and will do everything necessary to survive economically in the evolving dynamic health care and social enviornment. "It is important to recognize that we are not going to enjoy operating in isolation. We are going to be in the mainstream of what is going on nationally."

Acknowledging that Lorain is part of the delivery of health care services of nearby metropolitan Cleveland, he points out that "we will, for all practical purposes, be caught up in the Greater Cleveland synergy." In the complex interaction of many health care providers, the possibilities of expansions, reductions, networks, affiliations, and even closures of the various players must be examined frankly; hard decisions will be made, Balcom explains.

"What exactly these resolves will be may not be known in the immediate future. Within the next few years, as they become known, I think it will become self-evident that we will become enmeshed in collaboration, cooperation, or consolidated relationships with other hospitals and health care providers in our immediate as well as adjacent greater metropolitan Cleveland communities."

For three decades, Lorain Community Hospital has made serving and caring for its community its top priority. That will continue as the Board, Medical Staff, management, employees, and Auxiliary continue to dedicate their efforts to facing the challenges of the future.

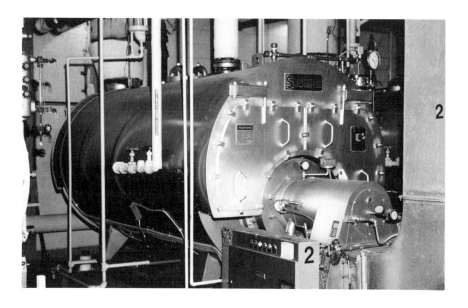

Environmental Services maintains equipment throughout the hospital for safety and maximum efficiency. Pictured here is the boiler room.

The Dream...The Journey
Lorain Community Hospital

1 9 9 2 L C H
F L O O R P L A N

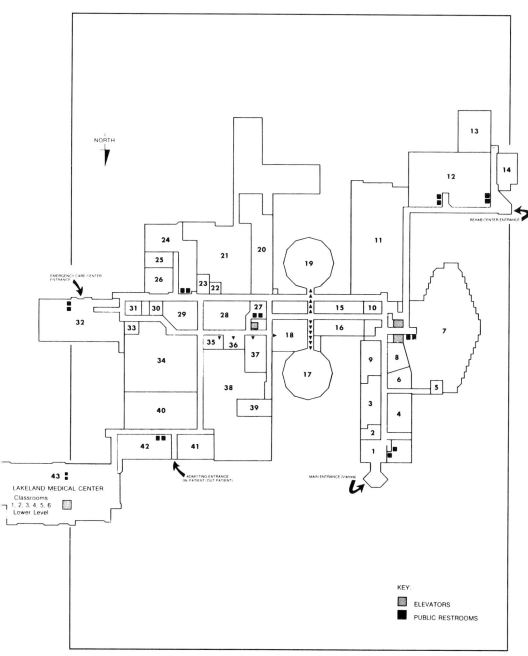

NORTH

REHAB CENTER ENTRANCE

EMERGENCY CARE CENTER ENTRANCE

ADMITTING ENTRANCE (IN-PATIENT-OUT PATIENT)

MAIN ENTRANCE (Visitors)

LAKELAND MEDICAL CENTER
Classrooms
1, 2, 3, 4, 5, 6
Lower Level

KEY:

ELEVATORS

PUBLIC RESTROOMS

DEPARTMENT DIRECTORY

17	I-NORTH (Patient Rooms 121-129)
19	I-SOUTH (Short Stay) (Patient Rooms 101-110)
7	I-WEST TOWER (Patient Rooms 163-195)
42	ADMITTING (Out-Patient)
36	AMBULATORY SURGI-CENTER
29	AUDITORIUM (David S. Ross)
3	BILLING OFFICE
28	BIO-MEDICAL
24	CAFETERIA (Lite House Cafe)
12	CARDIAC REHAB
3	CASHIER
31	CAST ROOM
30	CHAPEL
43	CLASSROOMS 1, 2, 3, 4, 5, 6 (Lakeland Medical Center)
26	CONFERENCE ROOM "A"
25	CONFERENCE ROOM "B"
23	CONFERENCE ROOM "C"
5	CONFERENCE ROOM "D"
6	CORKY'S (Sandwich Shop)
18	CRITICAL CARE CENTER (CCC)
32	EMERGENCY CARE CENTER (ECC)
9	EXECUTIVE OFFICE
35	FAMILY COUNSULTATION ROOM
27	FAMILY WAITING
13	GYM
37	INTENSIVE CARE CENTER (ICC)
40	LAB
2	LAKELAND HEALTH CARE (Physicians Billing)
43	LAKELAND MEDICAL CENTER (Classrooms 1, 2, 3, 4, 5, 6)
8	LIFE UNIFORM & SHOE (Treasure Chest)
24	LITE HOUSE CAFE (Cafeteria)
1	MAIN LOBBY
15	MEDICAL LIBRARY
4	MEDICAL RECORDS
16	NURSING ADMINISTRATION
21	NUTRITIONAL SERVICES
14	ORTHOPETIC PHYSICAL THERAPY
12	O.T. (Occupational Therapy) (Rehab Center)
41	PERSONNEL
12	P.T. (Physical Therapy) (Rehab Center)
2	PHYSICIANS BILLING (Lakeland Healthcare)
39	POST ANESTHESIA CARE UNIT (PACU) (Recovery)
39	RECOVERY (Post Anesthesia Care Unit) (PACU)
12	REHAB CENTER (O.T.) (P.T.)
20	REHAB SERVICES
6	SANDWICH SHOP (Corky's)
10	SECURITY (Lost & Found)
19	SHORT STAY (I-South) (Patient Rooms 101-110)
33	STRESS LAB
11	SPD (Supplies Processing & Distribution)
38	SURGERY
8	TREASURE CHEST (Life Uniform & Shoe)
22	VENDING
34	X-RAY

A P P E N D I X

MAJOR EVENTS IN THE HISTORY OF
LORAIN COMMUNITY HOSPITAL

1962   Ground-breaking for a 150-bed general hospital

1964   First patient admitted, ten beds available

1968   Coronary-care—intensive-care units become operational

1969   150-bed addition completed, 294 total registered beds

1972   Detoxification program initiated

        Emergency care center opened with Regional Poison Control Center designation

1975   Paul Balcom appointed Executive Director

1976   Formal Physician Recruitment program launched

        Physical medicine and rehabilitation services initiated

1977   *CT scanner installed

1979   Major facilities upgrade project undertaken. This included:

                Lakeland Medical Center (physician office building) opened on
                     hospital campus 1980

                Lakeland Institute Building (alcohol—chemical dependency) opened
                on hospital campus (first of two approved by state; fifty-bed
                     free-standing center)

                Digital subtraction angiography services initiated 1981

                Great Lakes Regional Rehabilitation Center—Comprehensive Physical
                     Medicine and Rehabilitation Services initiated 1982

                Urgent Care Center opened 1983

1981   Lakeland Guidance Centre (outpatient mental-health services) opened

1982   Regional Eye Center program formalized

1983   Parcourse opened

        *Hospital-based home health care program initiated

        *Level II trauma center developed and cited by American College of Surgeons as
                fully meeting college criteria

1984   Advanced level paramedic ground-rescue service initiated (dissolved in 1990)

        Pain Unit opened as part of Great Lakes Regional Rehabilitation program

        EAGLE (air-ambulance service) initiated (discontinued December 1985)

        Major corporate reorganization undertaken, including development of parent
                corporation; managed care company; for-profit entities, etc.

Appendix

1985   Lorain Community Hospital Foundation incorporated
        CT scanner upgrade completed
        Durable Medical Equipment Company formed (dissolved in 1989)
        Bond refinancing undertaken
1986   *Diabetes Comprehensive Care Center state-approved (formalization of an
                earlier developed service)
1987   Mammography suite opened
        Cardiac catheterization laboratory opened (following a four-year contested
                CON, including legal hearings and court proceedings)
1988   Expansion of Lakeland Medical Center begins (from 58,600 to
                99,338 square feet)
        Foundation capital campaign ("Saving Lives/Rebuilding Lives") undertaken
                ($2 million raised)
1989   Twenty-fifth Anniversary
        Regional Orthopedic Center dedicated
        Health information referral service introduced
        *Cleaver-Brooks multiple-chambered incinerator system, Model 780A, put in
                operation; state-of-the-art, EPA-approved for comprehensive, on-site
                incinerated waste disposal
1990   **Agreement with University Hospitals Network Affiliation consummated.
        Select Rehabilitation Services (industrial case management) launched
1991   Agreement with MedCenter Management for initiation of Center for Joint
                Implant Surgery consummated
        Formal total quality improvement program launched
1992   *Lakeland Institute 3/4-Way House program initiated
        *Hospital-based MRI services initiated
        *Stereotactic mammotest services offered
        Hospital maintains "A"-bond rating as it embarks on current revenue-bond
                refinancing
1993   *SNF (sixteen-bed, hospital-based, skilled nursing facility) opened

* First in Lorain County

**This relationship entered into in June, 1990 allowed LCH to be the first hospital in
Lorain County to enjoy a network membership with a tertiary care hospital.

Source: LCH report of organization's history

121

Edward W. Mehrer
1962—1965

Paul E. Friedlander
1966—1974

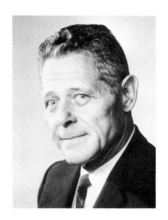

CHAIRMEN

OF

THE

BOARD

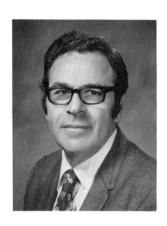

David S. Ross
1974—1984

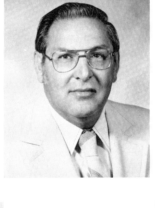

James L. Bardoner
1984—1992

Vincent P. Traina
1992—

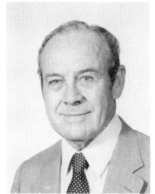

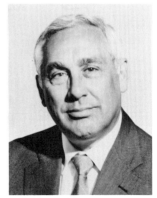

122

CHIEFS OF
MEDICAL STAFF

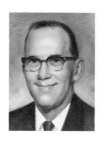 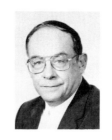

Robert P. Hardwig, M.D.
January 1, 1964—December 31, 1966
John J. Harrington, M.D. January 1,
1967—December 31, 1968

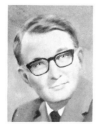 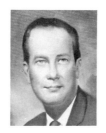 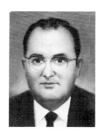 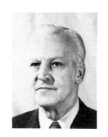

Raymond J. Py, M.D. January 1,
1969—June 1, 1969
John A. Grauel, M.D. June 1,
1969—September 1, 1969
John H. Paige, M.D. September 1,
1969—December 31, 1970
J. A. Dickason, M.D.
January 1, 1971—December 31, 1972

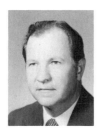 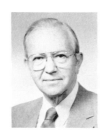 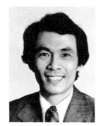 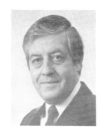

Peter A. Butrey, D.O.
January 1, 1973—December 31, 1974
Denis A. Radefeld, M.D.
January 1, 1975—December 31, 1978
Florencio Yuzon, M.D.
January 1, 1979—December 31, 1982
Stephan Ticich, M.D.
January 1, 1983—December 31, 1984

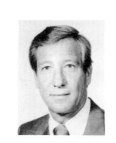 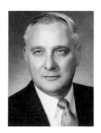 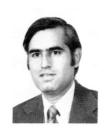

John Wright, M.D.
January 1, 1985—December 31, 1988
Donald Blanford, M.D.
January 1, 1989—December 31, 1992
Kumar Swamy, M.D.
January 1, 1993—

BOARD OF TRUSTEES 1993

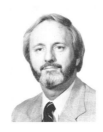 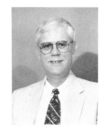 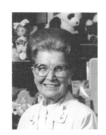
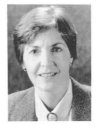 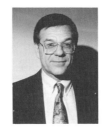 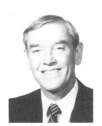
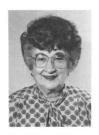 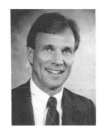 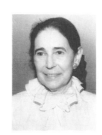
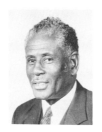

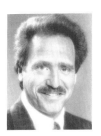 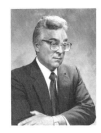 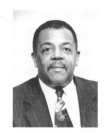

M. Orry Jacobs
Herman R. Kopf
William T. Locke

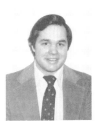 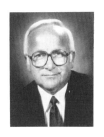 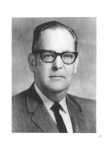

Stephen Meyer, M.D.
Stanley G. Pijor
Gerald L. Prucha

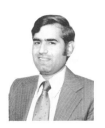 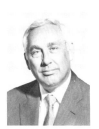 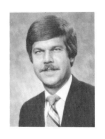

Kumar Swamy, M.D.
Vincent P. Traina
Richard L. Zahratka

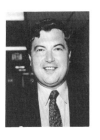 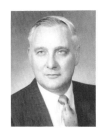

Alexander Zolli, M.D.
Donald Blanford, M.D.,
Ex Officio

CHIEF EXECUTIVE OFFICERS

James E. Huson, Administrator, November 1, 1963—May 8, 1968
Ross Garrett, Acting Administrator, May 8, 1968—September 9, 1968
    (title changed to Executive Director in June, 1968)
George O. West, Jr., Executive Director, September 9, 1968—June 1, 1975
Paul C. Balcom, Executive Director, June 1, 1975—
    (title changed to President and Chief Executive Officer in May 1987)

CHAIRMEN OF THE BOARD

Edward W. Mehrer 1962-65
Paul A. Friedlander 1966-74
David S. Ross 1974-84
James L. Bardoner 1984-92
Vincent P. Traina 1992-

LORAIN COMMUNITY HOSPITAL TRUSTEES
AND THEIR AFFILIATIONS
1964 TO 1993

Akins, John—Ford Motor Company
Amiri, M.A., M.D.—medical staff representative
Apolzon, George—Marathon Steel Products
Arnold, C. Marc—Ford Motor Company
Arora, P. Lal, M.D.—medical staff representative
Balcom, Paul C.—Lorain Community Hospital
Bardoner, James L.*—Dorn Industries (retired)
Bartek, Francis, M.D.—medical staff representative
Bescak, Kenneth, M.D.—medical staff representative

Bettcher, William H.—Bettcher Industries

Blanford, Donald, M.D.—chief of medical staff

Bobel, John—Bobel's Office Supply Products

Bohlmeyer, Frank G.—Cleveland Trust Bank

Bollin, Thomas D.—Lorain City Schools

Brandon, John, D.O.—medical staff representative

Bregman, Harold B.—Wagner Awning Company

Brugger, Gerold, M.D.—medical staff representative

Butrey, Peter, D.O.—chief of medical staff

Calta, Ruth—civic leader

Caprara, Albert J.—Ford Motor Company

Clark, John—Ford Motor Company

Conn, L. Wayne—Lorain Auto Parts Company

Corogin, Peter John—Lake Erie Electric, Inc.

Cromling, Maureen M.—Ross Environmental Services, Inc.

Danne, Howard E.—Ford Motor Company

DeLuca, Leonard—DeLuca's Place in the Park

Dickason, J. A., M.D.—chief of medical staff

Doane, Barbara—Auxiliary president

Dobrow, Estelle—Auxiliary president

Donnell, Frederick—Steel Stamping Company

Driscol, Paul E., Jr.—Driscol Music Company

Dziama, Marge—Auxiliary president

Faunt, Joseph R.

Finkel, Warren E.—Finkel & Finkel Architects

Fischer, Howard E.—Citizens Home & Savings Bank

Friedlander, Paul E.*—U.S. Steel Corporation

Full, Ray—Kishman Fish Company

Fusilero, Victorino, M.D.—medical staff representative

Grauel, John A., M.D.—chief of medical staff

Hageman, James C.—Lorain Telephone Company

Hardwig, Robert P., M.D.—chief of medical staff

Harrington, John, M.D.—chief of medical staff/medical staff representative

Hartley, Malcom D.—*The Lorain Journal*

Heiland, Kerwin D.—Ford Motor Company

Henry, James G.—Ford Motor Company

Herzer, Charles—American Crucible Products

Herzer, David L.—Wickens, Herzer & Panza Co., LPA

Hibbard, Robert—NASA

Hoke, Amalia V.—civic leader

Hunker, Jean—Auxiliary president

Inman, Fred—Ford Motor Company

Jackson, Clyde E.—UAW Local Union #425, Ford

Jacobs, M. Orry—University Hospitals of Cleveland Representative

Kantharaj, Belagodu, M.D.—medical staff representative

Kilmer, R. J.—Gregory Industries

Kingsley, Ross, D.O.—medical staff representative

Kopf, Herman R. "Bucky"—Kopf Construction Corporation

Laurence, R. L.

Locke, William T.—Lorain County Community Action Agency

Macgregor, Barbara—Auxiliary president

McGeachie, Thomas—Tom McGeachie Company

Martin, Thomas, M.D.—medical staff representative

Mehrer, Edward*—Ford Motor Company

Metzger, Madelyn—Auxiliary president

Meyer, Stephen, M.D.—medical staff representative

Meyers, Bristow, M.D.—Lorain physician

Nielsen, Carl G.—Nielsen Jewelers

Norton, Benjamin G., Jr.—Lorain Products

Obran, Frank J.—Labor Relations Representative, U.S. Steel Corporation

Paige, John, M.D.—chief of medical staff

Pashkevich, George—Labor Relations Representative, U.S. Steel Corporation

Patterson, James, M.D.—medical staff representative

Pelander, A. J.—City Bank Company

Pheiffer, John—Dorn Industries

Pijor, Stanley G.—Lorain National Bank, (Chair of LHCC —Holding
       Company for Hospital)

Prucha, Gerald L.—attorney at law

Py, Raymond J., M.D.—chief of medical staff

Radefeld, Denis A., M.D.—chief of medical staff

Rak, Wences—Labor Relations Representative, U.S. Steel Corporation

Restifo, Nicholas, D.O.—medical staff representative

Reynolds, Grace—civic leader

Riddell, James—Consumers Builders Supply Company

Ross, David S.*—Hydro-Clear Corporation

Roth, George L.—Roth Corporation

Rusin, Charlotte—auxiliary representative

Rusin, Conrad, M.D.—medical staff representative

Sanker, Ronald, D.O.—medical staff representative

Sedivy, Joseph F.—Labor Relations Representative, I.B.E.W.

Sfeir, Sami, M.D.—medical staff representative

Standen, Grace—The National Bank of Lorain

Steen, Elmer—U.S. Steel Corporation

Steen, Aleen (June)—Auxiliary president, honorary life member

Strippoli, Gino—TRW/Nelson Stud Welding Division

Swamy, Kumar, M.D.—medical staff representative/chief of medical staff

Swazin, John—U.S. Steel Corporation

Tellman, Annabel—Auxiliary president

Tharp, David, M.D.—medical staff representative

Ticich, Stephan, M.D.—chief of medical staff

Towner, Joyce J.—Auxiliary president

Traina, Vincent P.*—R.E. Warner & Associates, Inc.

Tyler, Janet—Auxiliary president

White, Terry R.—University Hospitals of Cleveland Representative

Wickens, William E.—Wickens & Wickens

Woodward, Robert I.—Woodward Construction Company

Wright, John, M.D.—chief of medical staff

Yuzon, Florencio, M.D.—chief of medical staff

Zahratka, Richard, CPA—Frank, Seringer & Chaney, Inc.

Zakowski, Charlotte—Auxiliary president

Ziegler, Richard—U.S. Steel Corporation
Zilka, Charles
Zolli, Alexander F., M.D.—medical staff representative

As of July 12, 1993
*Served as chairman of the Hospital Board of Trustees

LORAIN COMMUNITY HOSPITAL MEDICAL DIRECTORS

Denis A. Radefeld, M.D., 1986-1993
Donald B. Blanford, M.D., 1993-
Daniel C. Zaworksi, M.D., Assistant Medical Director, 1989-1993

Appendix

LORAIN COMMUNITY HOSPITAL
MEDICAL STAFF MEMBERS
APRIL 1964 TO SEPTEMBER 1993

Abella, D., M.D.
Abla, A., M.D.
Abramson, E., M.D.
Adamo, J., M.D.
Adams, C., M.D.
Adams, D., M.D.
Adams, G., D.O.
Adams, T., D.O.
Ahmed, I., M.D.
Alarcon, L., M.D.
Albanese, J., D.O.
Amiri, M., M.D.
Anderson, M., M.D.
Andrasko, J., M.D.
Armada, P., M.D.
Arnold, R., M.D.
Arora, P., M.D.
Aros, R., D.D.S.
Asuncion, L., M.D.
Athey, A., M.D.
Aycinena, P., M.D.
Bacevice, A., M.D.
Bacha, D., M.D.
Ball, E., M.D.
Ballis, S., M.D.
Balunek, A., M.D.
Barb, J., D.O.
Bartek, F., M.D.

Bartlett, J., D.O.
Bartulica, P., M.D.
Batizy, L., D.O.
Bear, P., D.O.
Beaver, B., D.O.
Belizaire, H., M.D.
Bentz, R., D.O.
Bentz, R., II, D.O.
Berkebile, R., M.D.
Berman, A., M.D.
Bescak, G., D.O.
Bescak, K., M.D.
Billowitz, A., M.D.
Biscardi, A., D.O.
Biscup, R., D.O.
Bitar, J., M.D.
Bittman, J., D.O.
Blackburn, J., D.O.
Blackman, S., M.D.
Blanford, D., M.D.
Bogoevski, V., M.D.
Boult, C., M.D.
Boye-Doe, A., M.D.
Brabender, W., M.D.
Bradley, K., M.D.
Brandon, J., D.O.
Brandon, M., D.O.
Bristow, M., M.D.

Brletic, J., D.D.S.
Brodsky, M., M.D.
Brucker, M., M.D.
Brugger, G., M.D.
Brugger, K., M.D.
Bukowski, M., M.D.
Burger, R., M.D.
Burma, G., M.D.
Burns, K., M.D.
Butrey, C., M.D.
Butrey, P., D.O.
Caldron, P., D.O.
Cann, J., D.P.M.
Cano, D., M.D.
Carandang, C., M.D.
Cardella, J., M.D.
Carney, J., M.D.
Castro, R., M.D.
Cayayan, N., M.D.
Chambers, J., D.O.
Chapla, A., M.D.
Chapple, C., M.D.
Chau, W., M.D.
Cherukuri, S., M.D.
Chesner, C., M.D.
Chohan, M., M.D.
Cicerrella, J., M.D.
Ciemins, A., M.D.

Cole-Sedivy, D., D.O.
Copperman, H., D.D.S.
Corzo-Moody, A., M.D.
Costin, J., M.D.
Cottle, J., D.D.S.
Cox, W., M.D.
Cragg, C., M.D.
Craven, P., M.D.
Cruz, T., M.D.
Cruz, W., M.D.
Cunningham, W., D.O.
Dacha, H., M.D.
Dacha, U., M.D.
Dakters, G., M.D.
D'Amico, L., M.D.
Darcy, K., M.D.
Darrow, J., M.D.
Davis, A., M.D.
Delaleu, S., M.D.
Dematte, C., D.D.S.
De Nardi, J., M.D.
Dengel, F., M.D.
Denny, K., M.D.
Derkash, R., M.D.
Diamond, R., D.O.
Diaz, R., M.D.
Dickason, J.H., M.D.
Dickason, J.R., M.D.
Dikranian, H., M.D.
DiVita, C., D.D.S.
Dobrow, D., M.D.
Doslak, W., D.D.S.
Duffy, D., D.P.M.

Drygas, H., M.D.
Edmunds, R., M.D.
Ellis, W., M.D.
Emdur, L, D.O.
Engstrom, C., M.D.
Eren, Ibrahim, M.D.
Eren, Itri, M.D.
Eren, M., M.D.
Escuro, R., M.D.
Espey, S., M.D.
Essel, E., M.D.
Essig, G., M.D.
Etzkorn, P., M.D.
Evans, D., D.O.
Evans, R., D.O.
Fanton, P., D.O.
Farhat, N., M.D.
Feicks, W., M.D.
Felski, E., D.O.
Ferber, W., M.D.
Fernando, R., M.D.
Ferrato, P., M.D.
Fildes, M,. M.D.
Fischer, D., M.D.
Flatt, D., M.D.
Flint, E., M.D.
Floro, F., M.D.
Fraley, E., M.D.
Frankle, H., M.D.
Froilan, J., M.D.
Furey, K., D.O.
Fusilero, V., M.D.
Gabarda, A., M.D.

Gaston, D., M.D.
Gencheff, N., D.O.
Gerber, E., M.D.
Gerson, S., M.D.
Ghanma, M., M.D.
Ghazi, F., M.D.
Gilman, I., D.D.S.
Gordillo, M., M.D.
Gossman, D., M.D.
Gotsis, G., M.D.
Graor, R., M.D.
Grauel, J., M.D.
Gray, J., D.O.
Grech, D., M.D.
Gressel, M., D.M.D.
Griffith, L., D.M.D.
Grigera, F., M.D.
Hait, L., M.D.
Haldeman, G., D.O.
Hale, R., M.D.
Hall, J., M.D.
Halley, J., M.D.
Hardwig, R., M.D.
Harms, G., M.D.
Harrington, J., M.D.
Hazen, G., M.D.
Hazen, M., M.D.
Hazen, P., M.D.
Heine, K., M.D.
Herberth, J., D.O.
Heyslinger, P., M.D.
Higgins, B., M.D.
Hoke, G., M.D.

Holden, D., M.D.

Holmes, R., M.D.

Horvitz, L., M.D.

Howren, P., D.O.

Hritz, M., M.D.

Huffman, K., D.O.

Hughes, M., M.D.

Huh, J., M.D.

Ingleright, B., D.O.

Irace, P., D.O.

Jacobs, K., M.D.

Jankas, R., D.P.M.

Jantsch, W., M.D.

Jarmoszuk, N., M.D.

Jasko, J., M.D.

Jenkins, C., M.D.

Jones, C., M.D.

Jones, K., D.O.

Jonesco, J., D.O.

Josef, D., M.D.

Joyce, D., M.D.

Judge, J., D.O.

Jung, Y., M.D.

Jurek, I., M.D.

Kantharaj, B., M.D.

Kata, J., D.O.

Kavuru, M., M.D.

Kearney, F., M.D.

Keiser, H., M.D.

Keller, J., D.O.

Keller, J., D.P.M.

Kent, D., M.D.

Keppler, L., M.D.

Kherani, R., M.D.

Kilmer, T., D.O.

Kingsley, R., D.O.

Kishman, W., M.D.

Kleinhenz, H., M.D.

Klimas, P., M.D.

Kohn, M., M.D.

Kolczun, M., I, M.D.

Kolczun, M., II, M.D.

Kooba, E., M.D.

Korbol, M., D.P.M.

Korinek, J., M.D.

Kramer, K., M.D.

Kreindel, M., M.D.

Krishnan, T., M.D.

Krupp, G., M.D.

Krupski, J., M.D.

Lai, Y., M.D.

Lampl, B., D.O.

Langston, R., M.D.

LaRiccia, L., D.O.

Lawrence, C., D.O.

Lee, D., M.D.

Lehnowsky, R., D.D.S.

Lenhart, R., M.D.

Leone, D., M.D.

Leslie, S., M.D.

Levine, M., M.D.

Lindgren, P., D.D.S.

Linstruth, K., M.D.

Liu, A., D.O.

Loser, A., M.D.

Love, C. Jackson, D.D.S.

Love, C. James, D.D.S.

Lumanlan, A., M.D.

McCoy, J., M.D.

McGuinn, W., M.D.

Macchi, M., M.D.

Mace, S., M.D.

Mahajan, D., M.D.

Maher, J., M.D.

Mahilo, J., D.D.S.

Mandel, D., M.D.

Marek, J., M.D.

Marfori, N., M.D.

Marks, R., M.D.

Marquart, J., M.D.

Marr, L., M.D.

Marr, V., M.D.

Martin, T., M.D.

Martinez, E., M.D.

Martinez, L., M.D.

Martinez, Z., M.D.

Mattey, A., M.D.

Matysik, G., M.D.

May, F., M.D.

Mazorow, H., D.D.S.

Meany, F., M.D.

Meckler, J., D.D.S.

Mehta, A., M.D.

Mehta, G., M.D.

Meimaridis, S., M.D.

Meyer, S., M.D.

Mick, M., M.D.

Miclat, R., M.D.

Mikhail, M., M.D.

Miller, C., M.D.	O'Shaughnessy, C., M.D.	Restifo, N., D.O.
Miranda, F., M.D.	Ostrum, A., D.O.	Ridley, D., M.D.
Miyara, A., M.D.	Ozbardakci, D., M.D.	Ringel, R., M.D.
Moon, T., M.D.	Padilla, C., M.D.	Rittenour, R., D.O.
Moore, S., D.D.S.	Paige, J., M.D.	Rivera, J., M.D.
Moore, S., D.O.	Parikh, S., M.D.	Robalino, B., M.D.
Mora, R., M.D.	Patel, C., M.D.	Rooney, T., D.O.
Moroni, R., M.D.	Patel, D., M.D.	Rosario, A., M.D.
Morris, R., M.D.	Patel, K., M.D.	Rosenbaum, H., M.D.
Mostow, N., M.D.	Patterson, F., M.D.	Rosevear, M., M.D.
Mota, F., M.D.	Patterson, J., M.D.	Rusin, C., M.D.
Mourad, S., M.D.	Patterson, V., M.D.	Russell, D., M.D.
Mulford, R., D.O.	Pecorak, J., M.D.	Sabga, G., M.D.
Mullin, T., M.D.	Peebles, T., M.D.	Safi, B., M.D.
Munoz, F., M.D.	Pena, Carlos, M.D.	Salka, M., M.D.
Myers, B., M.D.	Pena, Cesar, M.D.	Samtoy, B., M.D.
Naeem, S., M.D.	Piechal, W., D.O.	Sanchez, C., M.D.
Nazarian, L., M.D.	Pietrolungo, J., M.D.	Sandigo, J., M.D.
Nedorost, S., M.D.	Plank, T., D.O.	Sandoval, V., M.D.
Neff, F., M.D.	Plas, J., M.D.	Sanker, R., D.O.
Nemeth, V., M.D.	Polinski, W., D.O.	Sauder, H., M.D.
Nepomuceno, O., M.D.	Powell, G., D.O.	Scarcella, J., M.D.
Newdow, M., M.D.	Price, J., M.D.	Schaeffer, J., M.D.
Nguyen, T., D.O.	Prior, M., M.D.	Schechtman, J., D.O.
Novello, A., M.D.	Py, R., M.D.	Schneer, R., M.D.
Novello, J., M.D.	Quan, W., M.D.	Schotz, R., M.D.
Noveske, G., M.D.	Raczak, A., M.D.	Schwert, R., M.D.
Oberer, K., D.O.	Radefeld, D., M.D.	Sciarrotta, J., M.D.
O'Campo, T., M.D.	Ralston, W., M.D.	Secrist, J., M.D.
Oey, H., M.D.	Read, M., M.D.	Segarra, S., M.D.
Oh, P., D.O.	Rebchook, A., M.D.	Seng, M., M.D.
Ohliger, J., D.O.	Reed, W., M.D.	Seo, J., M.D.
Olin, J., D.O.	Reisman, J., M.D.	Serrano, J., M.D.

Sertich, M., M.D.
Sfeir, S., M.D.
Sfiligoj, T., M.D.
Shapiro, D., M.D.
Sharbek, M., M.D.
Sheldon, D., M.D.
Sheldon, W., M.D.
Shor, S., M.D.
Shultz, Kelley, M.D.
Sigalove, W., M.D.
Silecky, J., M.D.
Silver, T., M.D.
Sisam, D., D.O.
Sison, D., M.D.
Smead, H., M.D.
Smit, J., M.D.
Smith, T., M.D.
Snell, E., M.D.
Sokovs, I., M.D.
Stanbro, M., D.O.
Stevens, R., D.O.
Stewart, J., M.D.
Stout, D., M.D.
Suico, E., M.D.
Suico, V., M.D.
Sun, Y., M.D.
Swamy, K., M.D.
Sym, J., M.D.
Szentendrey, K., M.D.
Tabaie, H., D.O.
Taylor, L., M.D.
Taylor, W., D.O.
Thompson, M., D.O.

Thorley, L., M.D.
Ticich, S., M.D.
Toledo, J., M.D.
Torelli, J., M.D.
Treuhaft, P., M.D.
Trzeciak, A., M.D.
Trzeciak, V., M.D.
Turowski, J., D.O.
Vacante, M., D.O.
Van Bergen, R., M.D.
Vanek, J., M.D.
Varley, P., M.D.
Vassilakis, G., M.D.
Villa, A., M.D.
Von Kaenel, W., M.D.
Waddell, J., D.P.M.
Wagner, W., D.O.
Watson, L., D.O.
Weimken, G., D.P.M.
Weiner, K., D.O.
Welch, G., D.O.
Wendschuch, P., M.D.
Whitted, G., M.D.
Wilber, J., M.D.
Wilber, R., M.D.
Wilke, R., M.D.
Williams, T., M.D.
Wiseman, G., M.D.
Witcik, W., M.D.
Woisnet, T., M.D.
Woodward, R., M.D.
Wright, J., M.D.
Wright, R., M.D.

Yepko, H., D.D.S.
Yood, C., M.D.
Young, W., M.D.
Yu, M., M.D.
Yusufaly, I., M.D.
Yuzon, F., M.D.
Zantua, A., M.D.
Zaworski, D., M.D.
Zaylor, R., M.D.
Zbornik, R., M.D.
Zegarra, H., M.D.
Zelenski, J., D.O.
Zelenski, S., D.O.
Zgrabik, M., M.D.
Zolli, A., M.D.

LORAIN COMMUNITY HOSPITAL AUXILIARY PRESIDENTS

1964-66   Amalia (Laurie) Hoke
1967-68   Aleen June Steen
1969-70   Grace Reynolds
1971-72   Ruth Calta
1973-74   Annabel Tellman
1975-76   Barbara Doane
1977-78   Joyce J. Towner
1979-80   Madelyn Metzger
1981-82   Janet Tyler
1983-84   Barbara Macgregor
1985-86   Charlotte Zakowski
1987   Janet Tyler
1988   Barbara Macgregor
1989-91   Estelle Dobrow
1991-93   Jean Hunker
1993-   Marge Dziama

Source: LCH Auxiliary Handbook for Adult Volunteers, 1993